Time to Go

Time to Go

Three Plays on Death and Dying
with Commentary on End-of-Life Issues

Edited by
Anne Hunsaker Hawkins, Ph.D. and
James O. Ballard, M.D.
with
Theodore Blaisdell, M.D.

University of Pennsylvania Press

Philadelphia

The University of Pennsylvania Press will grant permission for performance of the plays in *Time to Go* only on the condition that performances will be free of charge. Parties requesting that this condition be waived must secure written permission from the author of the play in question, who can be contacted c/o the University of Pennsylvania Press.

Copyright © 1995 by the Doctors Kienle Center for Humanistic Medicine
All rights reserved
Printed in the United States of America

Library of Congress Cataloging-in-Publication Data
    Time to go: three plays on death and dying, with commentary on end-of-life issues /
edited by Anne Hunsaker Hawkins and James O. Ballard with Theodore Blaisdell.
        p.   cm.
    Includes bibliographical references and index.
    Contents: Journey into that good night / Berry L. Barta — Stars at the break of day /
Marjorie Ellen Spence — Time to go / CE McClelland.
    ISBN 0-8122-1519-2
    1. Death — Drama.   2. Do-not-resuscitate orders — Drama.   3. American drama — 20th
century.   4. Right to die — Drama.   I. Hawkins, Anne Hunsaker, 1944–   .   II. Ballard,
James O.   III. Blaisdell, Theodore.
PS627.D42T56   1995
306.9 — dc20   94-32201
                                                                                                       CIP

Dedicated to the memory of
JANE WITMER KIENLE, M.D.

Contents

The Introduction was written by James O. Ballard, with Anne Hunsaker Hawkins adding the concluding section. Commentaries on all three plays were written by Hawkins. Suggestions for staging and discussion are the work of Hawkins and Theodore Blaisdell. Ballard compiled the appendices.

Acknowledgments

Many people have made generous contributions to the development of this book and the project on which it is based. No contribution, however, could be more important than that of Lawrence F. Kienle and Jane Witmer Kienle. The Doctors Kienle Center for Humanistic Medicine not only funded the script-writing contest that yielded the plays in this book, but also subsidized the book's publication.

The Kienle Center began as The Center for Humanistic Medicine of the Milton S. Hershey Medical Center in 1979, founded through the joint efforts of the departments of Humanities, Medicine, and Behavioral Science. Its mission was—and still is—to support, facilitate, and initiate education and research that will render the delivery of health care more humane, both locally and nationally. It was in 1985, when Dr. Jane Witmer Kienle (a retired psychiatrist) and Dr. Lawrence F. Kienle (a retired radiologist) joined The Center as benefactors, that it really began to thrive. The Kienles were looking for an institution which would support the advancement of humanistic medical values, and it is our great good fortune that they found Hershey and its Center for Humanistic Medicine, which has been transformed by their generous backing. The Center now includes representatives from eighteen different departments and supports many educational and research projects that concern humane medical practice. With the sudden death of Jane Kienle, to whom this book is dedicated, we lost a dear friend. However, Larry has worked tirelessly to see that the entire scope of Jane's and his vision for The Center would be realized. A new era began in 1992, when a generous additional gift led The Center to be renamed "The Doctors Kienle Center for Humanistic Medicine."

This book illustrates the goals and work of The Kienle Center: to advance the partnership of medical professionals, patients, and the community in fostering the most effective and compassionate medical care possible. It is the position of The Kienle Center that, during this period of medical reform, nothing is more crucial than maintaining the connection between technical excellence and humane values in care. We hope that our book will serve this purpose.

The editors wish to thank Sherman Hawkins, professor emeritus at Wesleyan University, for his many contributions to our medical theater project. We are also grateful to Ted Blaisdell, a fine physician as well as a superb actor and director; Russell Miller, founding member and student organizer of the Hershey Medical Theater Group; Robert Biter, talented actor, director, and playwright, who succeeds Miller as HMTG student organizer; and all the medical students, physicians, staff, and their spouses who served as actors in our plays.

We are grateful for permission to use copyrighted material in several instances. William Carlos Williams's, "The Red Wheelbarrow," in *The Collected Works of William Carlos Williams, 1909–1939,* vol. 1, copyright © 1938 New Directions Publishing Corporation, is used by permission of New Directions Publishing Corporation. An excerpt from W. H. Auden's "Musée des Beaux Arts," in *W. H. Auden: Collected Poems,* ed. Edward Mendelson, copyright © 1940, renewed 1968 by W. H. Auden, is reprinted by permission of Random House. An excerpt from Dylan Thomas's "Do Not Go Gentle into That Good Night" is reprinted by permission of Harry Ober Associates, Random House, Inc., and Alfred E. Knopf, Inc. "The Values History" (Appendix A), an excerpt from David J. Doukas and L. B. McCullough, "The Values History: The Evaluation of the Patient's Values and Advance Directives," *Journal of Family Practice* 32 (1991): 145–53, copyright © 1991, is reprinted by permission of the authors, the *Journal of Family Practice,* and Appleton and Lange Publishers. The model documents contained in Appendix B and Appendix C are reprinted by permission of the American Association of Retired Persons.

Part I

Advance Directives: Starting the Dialogue

Introduction

The Problem

In our country's health care institutions, decisions are made every day regarding the use of life-sustaining medical treatment. It is estimated that 80 percent of deaths occur in a hospital or nursing home setting, and that for 70 percent of these individuals a decision is made either not to start or to terminate medical therapy.[1] This scenario is all too familiar to health care workers. A patient with a prior diagnosis of advanced lung disease, metastatic cancer, or AIDS is readmitted to the hospital complaining of severe shortness of breath. Things go from bad to worse, and an urgent decision must be made whether mechanical ventilation will be initiated. The patient is now too ill to comprehend and participate in decision making.

The patient and physician may have had a mutual understanding that the long-term prognosis of the underlying disease process is not good, but the two have not discussed what the patient would want done or not done in the current situation. The physician may have reason to believe this new complication is reversible, but at the same time there is a painful awareness that the patient may remain dependent on the ventilator, even if the underlying lung infection is resolved.

The family is divided, with some members urging the doctor to "Do everything possible"; others saying, "Just make him comfortable"; and yet others, "Do what you think is best." Furthermore, the physician may even fear legal action if he or she withholds or terminates life support.

The site where these end-of-life decisions are made may compound the problem. Patients with life-threatening illnesses such as those depicted above are frequently sent to tertiary care medical centers, with the understanding and hope that they will receive the latest and best treatment available. The "best" treatment has come to mean highly technical and costly therapy that has the potential of sustaining life indefinitely by mechanical and pharmacologic means. In these medical centers, not one but several physicians, nurses, and other health care providers are responsible for assessing and treating the patient. As the complexity of the patient's problems increases, specialists are called in and each makes recommendations from his or her particular area of expertise — but not necessarily with an understanding of the patient's life history or the overall plan of care for this patient.

Thus it may become difficult to distinguish the patient from the technology and hard to identify the individual who is in charge of making medical decisions for the patient. The real tragedy of this situation is that, in the absence of written or verbal instructions from the patient, it is impossible to ensure that the patient's wishes are being followed. It is also quite likely that the patient would not have wanted to subject his or her family to the emotional upheaval inherent in grappling with a decision to withhold or terminate life support.

Historical Background

The historical underpinning of the recent national focus on advance planning begins with the basic rights of privacy guaranteed by common, state and constitutional law. In 1914, Judge Benjamin Cardozo of New York wrote in *Schloendorff v. New York Hospital:*

> Every human being of adult years and sound mind has a right to determine what shall be done with his own body and cannot be subjected to medical treatment without his consent.[2]

In 1928, Supreme Court Justice Louis Brandeis elaborated on this theme, and his statements have influenced subsequent court decisions regarding the essential right to refuse medical treatment. He wrote concerning the intent of the framers of the U.S. Constitution that they "conferred, as against the Government, the right to be let alone — the most comprehensive of rights and the right most valued by civilized men."[3]

Following World War II and continuing to the present, there has been a remarkable transformation of American health care. The number of hospitals in this country increased dramatically in the 1950s and, along with this, the locus of care changed from the home and physician's office to medical institutions. In the 1960s through the 1980s, new drugs, government-sponsored medical research, and advances in medical technology began to revolutionize health care in ways not previously imagined.

The doctrine of informed consent signaled that a gradual change in the fundamental relationship between health care provider and patient was taking place. Jay Katz chronicles the evolution of the doctrine of informed consent,[4] beginning with the 1957 case of Martin Salgo, a 55-year-old man who developed lower extremity paralysis following an arterial injection of dye for an X-ray study. Mr. Salgo first claimed that the paralysis resulted from negligent performance of the arterial injection, and he later also maintained that the physician performing the study had failed to warn him of the risk of paralysis before beginning the procedure. In his pronouncements on this case, Justice Bray of the California Court of Appeals coined the phrase "informed consent" to describe the process by which patients are given all the facts required to enable them to make a knowledgeable decision whether to allow or to refuse a proposed treatment.

In the landmark cases of *Natanson v. Kline* in 1960 and *Canterbury v. Spence* in 1972,[5] the right of an individual to receive full disclosure prior to giving consent for procedures and medical treatments was reaffirmed; however, the decisions in these two cases articulated a dilemma, namely, how much should the physician tell the patient? Would full disclosure of the risks hinder the patient's acceptance of potentially life-saving therapy, or would it somehow cause psychological damage to the individual? Justice Schroeder in *Natanson v. Kline* voiced this concern:

> There is probably a privilege, on therapeutic grounds, to withhold the specific diagnosis where the disclosure of cancer or some dread disease would seriously jeopardize the recovery of an unstable, temperamental or severely depressed patient.

Today, the moral and legal grounds for the full disclosure of diagnosis and treatment effects are widely accepted by physicians. However, the tension between complete and truthful disclosure, on the one hand, and the concern that this information might pose a risk to the patient's well-being, on the other, is still problematic for some physicians and families.

The widespread use of the mechanical respirator and the development of the techniques of cardiopulmonary resuscitation (CPR) and artificial nutrition allowed prolongation of life for patients with potentially reversible medical conditions. Since some individuals resuscitated by these treatments never regained consciousness but could have their breathing and cardiac activity maintained indefinitely by artificial means, new ethical problems surfaced.

In 1976, California became the first state to pass laws allowing people to declare their wishes for life-sustaining treatment in documents that would go into effect if they became seriously ill and unable to communicate. The same year, the storm surrounding patient self-determination began gaining momentum in New Jersey with the case of Karen Ann Quinlan. Quinlan had suffered two episodes during which blood flow to the brain had been compromised, leaving her in a persistent vegetative state — a condition of eyes-open, permanent unconsciousness in which a person retains some involuntary motor reflexes but loses all cognitive function. Her parents sought court authorization to remove her from a respirator. The New Jersey Supreme Court voted unanimously to authorize removal of mechanical ventilation on the basis of a constitutional right of privacy, which the court argued would be lost unless the family were allowed to exercise the right on her behalf.[6]

Over the next fifteen years, courts in twenty states heard cases regarding treatment for patients who were "incompetent" to make health care decisions, that is, were determined to lack the ability to comprehend and act upon information provided. In these cases, the right of *competent* individuals to forgo medical treatment was upheld. Furthermore, most state courts authorized surrogate decision making for *incompetent* patients. The notable exceptions were New York[7] and Missouri.

The Missouri case *Cruzan v. Harmon*[8] has become the single most important case regarding termination of life support. Nancy Beth Cruzan, a young woman in a persistent vegetative state as a result of an automobile accident, required only a feeding tube to continue to survive. By 1988, she had remained permanently unconscious for approximately five years and had continued to receive feedings and water by a gastric tube.

Her parents firmly believed she would not want tube feedings continued under such circumstances — a belief based in part on their remembrance of her comment that she would not want to live if she could not be "at least halfway normal." In 1988 Mr. and Mrs. Cruzan sought and received court authorization for removal of the feeding tube. The hospital staff caring for Ms. Cruzan refused to obey the order to terminate artificial nutrition, and the Missouri Supreme Court reversed the decision of the lower court. The Missouri Supreme Court held that no one except Nancy Cruzan could exercise her right to refuse treatment, since the consequence of this refusal would be death, and that the state had a primary interest in preserving the life of its citizens unless there was "clear and convincing evidence" that she herself had rejected the treatment.[9]

The U.S. Supreme Court upheld Missouri's decision to adopt a standard of clear and convincing evidence, but at the same time it strongly affirmed that all *competent* persons have a "liberty interest" to refuse life-sustaining therapy. Following this, in 1990, the Missouri courts found that there was, in fact, clear and convincing evidence of the patient's desire to be allowed to die. The gastric tube was removed, and Nancy Cruzan died ten days later.[10]

The Patient Self-Determination Act

The Quinlan and Cruzan cases illustrate how medical technology has dramatically altered the practice of medicine and how the context in which people die has also changed. Prior to the 1950s, there was little that could be done to prolong life. People frequently died at home under the watchful care of a physician who had known the patient for years. Today, the last physicians to care for a patient before death may have known the patient for only a brief time. The need to initiate life-sustaining medical treatment is likely to arise as a crisis situation and at a point when there is insufficient time to weigh the benefits and burdens of a given form of therapy. It is against this background that the Patient Self-Determination Act (PSDA) emerged.

Sponsored by Senator John Danforth (R-MO) and Senator Patrick Moynihan (D-NY), the PSDA became law as part of the Omnibus Budget Reconciliation Act of 1990,[11] which had the overall goal of keeping the federal government financially solvent. A stated goal of the PSDA is to ensure a patient's right to participate in and help direct health care decisions.

The PSDA requires that, beginning in December 1991, all medical facilities that accept Medicare and Medicaid payments (including hospitals, skilled nursing facilities, home health agencies, hospice organizations and HMOs) provide written information to patients about their rights under state law to make decisions about their medical care. Such decisions include the right to accept or refuse medical treatment and to complete advance medical directives such as a *living will* or *durable power of attorney for health care decisions*. The primary provisions of the PSDA require the provider institution to do the following:

- On admission, inform all patients of "an individual's rights under state law (whether statutory or as recognized by the courts of the state) to make decisions concerning such medical care, including the right to accept or refuse medical or surgical treatment and the right to formulate advance directives" and the right to receive summaries of "the written policies of the provider organization respecting the implementation of such rights."

- Document in the individual's medical record whether or not the individual has executed an advance medical directive.
- Not condition the provision of care or otherwise discriminate against an individual based on whether or not the individual has executed an advance directive.
- Ensure compliance with state law.
- Provide for education for staff and community on issues concerning advance directives.

Thus the intent of the PSDA is to increase public awareness of advance directives and to encourage people to examine their own values and preferences regarding the kind of medical treatment they would or would not want at the end of life. The great hope of the PSDA is that individuals will begin thinking about and executing advance directives long before the time when they might actually need these documents to direct their own health care. The PSDA can in fact be considered "community education legislation."[12]

An Assessment of Values

Before individuals can complete a legal document directing others to act on their behalf in making decisions about terminal medical care, they must clarify their own underlying beliefs and values. A key question that needs to be answered is "What kind of medical condition, if any, would make life so hard for me that attempts to prolong my life would be undesirable?" Also fundamental to this assessment is the weighing of the relative importance of length of life versus quality of life, as contained in such statements as: "I want to live as long as possible, regardless of the quality of life that I experience" versus "I want to preserve a good quality of life, even if this means that I may not live as long."[13]

David Doukas and Laurence McCullough have developed a "Values History" (see Appendix A) to serve as a starting point in discussions about personal values relevant to end-of-life decisions. For some individuals, the most important goal of terminal care will be a respect for their dignity and an assurance of physical and emotional comfort; for others, it might be the desire to be treated in accordance with their religious and philosophical beliefs. It is important that an individual's family, physician, and any designated decision makers be fully aware of these expressions of personal values and preferences so that they can help make informed decisions for the patient when the need arises.

Advance Directives: Expressing Values and Preferences in Writing

It is essential at the outset to recognize that any expression of preference for or against life-prolonging measures, whether verbal or writtten, has legal significance. To state this another way, written advance directives better ensure that patients' rights that already exist under common law and constitutional law will be acknowledged. When an individual becomes incompetent to make treatment decisions, he or she does not lose these common law and constitutional rights; the problem becomes one of determining the specific treatment preferences of that individual.[14]

Most states have enacted statutes that endorse two types of written documents for directing medical treatment decisions — the *living will* and the *durable power of attorney for health care*. In these states, advance directives can be executed by any competent person who is at least eighteen years of age or an "emancipated minor" (that is, who is a high school graduate or who has married). Advance directives have two major benefits: they help ensure that a person's wishes regarding medical care at the end of life will be honored, and they help protect family, friends, and physicians from the stress and potential conflict that can arise when there is an incomplete understanding of the patient's values and preferences. A person may elect to execute either or both types of document. Each has its merits and drawbacks, and if executed together, the two documents can complement each other.

Although variable from state to state, the *living will* gives specific directions about health care to be followed when two conditions are met: (1) the patient has a terminal illness or is permanently unconscious; and (2) the patient has become incapacitated. The definition of "terminal illness" differs from state to state, but in general, the condition must be an irreversible one that will lead to death within a defined time frame. Many states add the phrase "with or without life-sustaining treatment." The term "capacity" and its legal equivalent, "competent," are frequently used inter-changeably to define the capability to make decisions as: (1) the ability to comprehend information relevant to the decision; (2) the ability to deliber-ate about choices in accordance with personal values and goals; and (3) the ability to communicate (verbally and nonverbally) with care givers.[15]

The living will need not be complex and can follow a format such as that suggested by the American Association of Retired Persons (see Appen-dix B). Usually the directive begins with a statement that, if death is imminent, the process of dying should not be prolonged, but that all care should be directed at ensuring patient comfort and dignity. Some model documents then permit individuals to specify medical treatments they would or would not desire at this point in their lives. This might include interventions such as CPR, during which chest compression and/or elec-tric shock are used to attempt to restore heartbeat; mechanical ventilation, that is, machine-assisted breathing using a tube inserted in the trachea; kidney dialysis; surgery; artificial nutrition by a gastric tube; and other forms of supportive care.[16]

All states with living will statutes require that they be signed by at least two adult witnesses, and some states stipulate that one or both witnesses not be relatives or persons who might inherit the patient's estate, individ-uals who have financial responsibility for the patient's health care, or profes-sionals in charge of the patient's care. A lawyer is not required for the execution of an advance directive, but in some states the document must be notarized.

As of May 1994, forty-seven states and the District of Columbia had living will statutes. The three states which had not enacted living will legislation at this time are Massachusetts, Michigan, and New York.

Shortcomings of living wills include that they cannot provide guidance for circumstances not anticipated at the time the will was written, and that they usually apply only in the context of a terminal illness or condition of permanent unconsciousness. Also, they can be misplaced and are of no use unless others — family, designated health care proxy, and physician — know of their existence.

All state jurisdictions have generic durable power of attorney statutes, and most states now have specific laws governing health care power of attorney. This second type of advance directive, the *durable power of attorney for health care (DPA)*, is a written document in which a person designates an agent or "proxy" to make health care decisions in the event he or she becomes incapacitated. The DPA is considered a more flexible instrument than the living will for several reasons. (1) It allows the agent to make medical decisions for the patient in situations that could not have been anticipated at the time the living will was completed; that is, the proxy can weigh those benefits and burdens that are relevant for the patient at a specific point in time. (2) It applies to all medical decisions (unless limitations are imposed by the patient), not just those made in the context of a terminal illness. (3) It can include specific instructions for the agent to follow.

A DPA is not difficult to create and can follow a published model form such as that recommended by the American Association of Retired Persons (see Appendix C). The "attorney-of-fact" for health care decisions designated by the patient can be anyone — family member, friend, clergy, lawyer — whom the patient trusts to apply his or her values to the specific decision at hand. It is recommended that more than one agent be named and that, because of potential conflicts of interest, health care professionals and employees of health care facilities should *not* be named. The DPA must be witnessed and notarized as indicated by state law. Although not all states require notarization, the document should nevertheless be notarized so that it can be used in any state where the individual may travel or reside.

The advance directive statutes of individual states differ in their format and requirements. The most significant variations among state living will legislation include: (1) whether the statute applies to individuals in a persistent vegetative state and those with irreversible coma; (2) the extent to which the state statute permits the withholding of artificial nutrition and hydration; and (3) the application of advance directives for life-prolonging therapy for pregnant women. It is therefore important to be aware of the specific requirements of the state where the documents will be created and used. Appendix D lists resources for state-specific information on advance directives, which can be obtained from organizations such as the American Bar Association and Choice in Dying.

Barriers to Dialogue About Advance Directives

One of the important unstated benefits of the PSDA is that of encouraging conversation about preferences for future medical care. The principal participants in this discussion are the patient, the physician, and the family. It seems likely that in the future, society — in its role as guardian of health care resources — will assume a larger share in this dialogue. Although issues such as incompetence, terminal illness, and death are not easy to talk about, research studies indicate that both patients and the general public are eager to have these conversations regarding future treatment.[17] A study conducted in Boston in the late 1980s indicated that 93 percent of outpatients in primary care practices and 89 percent of the general public said they wanted one or more forms of advance directives. Furthermore, this study found that specific treatment preferences could not be predicted on the basis of age, current health status, or other demographic characteristics of the study population.[18]

By comparison, in a 1988 questionnaire study of attitudes regarding advance directives, conducted among a large group of Arkansas physicians practicing general medicine, family medicine, and internal medicine, approximately 89 percent of those polled agreed or strongly agreed with the statement that "advance directives are an effective way for patients to influence their medical treatment should they lose competence."[19] Perceived positive benefits of treatment directives for these physicians' patients included less patient anxiety, facilitation of physician-family agreement, a more trusting relationship, and a decrease in the tendency to practice "defensive medicine" for fear of malpractice suits.

The PSDA mandates that, on admission to medical institutions receiving Medicare or Medicaid funds, patients be provided with information about their rights to refuse treatment and to execute advance directives. In the time period from January to September 1992, a total of 2,134 patients were admitted to the University Hospitals of the Milton S. Hershey Medical Center in Hershey, Pennsylvania. Of these patients only 15 percent had completed a living will or designated a health care proxy, and of those without an advance directive, only 15 percent accepted referrals to social service or pastoral care to learn more about advance planning.[20] This experience seems to be similar to that reported elsewhere.[21] Although there appears to be widespread support for advance directives among patients, physicians, and the general public, only a minority of people have actually executed these documents and most choose to put off discussing the issue. Why should this be so?

L. L. Emanuel et al., in their survey of outpatients and the general public, found that the major barrier to executing a medical directive was not the disturbing nature of thinking about terminal illness and death, but rather (1) the expectation that the physician should take the initiative and (2) a perception that these are issues relevant for individuals who were older or in worse health.[22]

Other concerns about advance directives, on the part of both the public and physicians, have been summarized in the medical literature.[23] In general, most of these concerns reflect our natural inclination to procrastinate, rationalized by doubts that any directive completed in advance of a crisis could truly reflect the wishes of individuals at the time they are facing death. Some physicians are concerned that a discussion of advance directives early in the course of an illness may rob patients of a sense of hope in their prescribed treatment and confidence in their physician. Others worry that an advance directive is not flexible enough to allow for the changes that occur in a patient's medical condition over time. L. L. Emanuel and Ezekiel J. Emanuel have attempted to overcome some of the limitations of the conventional advance directive format. They have proposed a novel and comprehensive advance directive document[24] that asks individuals to make decisions about life-sustaining treatment by considering four case scenarios depicting actual illness circumstances involving mental incompetence. Their model document also allows for a proxy designation and a decision regarding organ donation.

Aside from these concerns and attempts at their solution, it seems that physicians and patients find it difficult to set aside the time necessary to talk with each other about advance directives. In an ideal world, a physician should initiate a discussion about advance planning with each adult patient as part of the initial evaluation and treatment plan, and then revisit and revise the directive at intervals along the course of the patient's illness. If the physician were to find that he or she could not in good conscience carry out the patient's directive, the patient should be so informed, and should then be assisted in selecting another physician who is willing to carry out the directive. In the real world, however, it seems that most individuals wait for their physician to initiate a discussion about advance planning, while at the same time physicians wait for signals that their patient is ready to talk about these matters.

Community and medical staff education can help the public and their physicians deal with the anxieties surrounding the issues of incapacity, terminal illness, and death. The physician-patient relationship has been characterized as being too frequently a silent partnership.[25] Truthful disclosure of diagnosis and prognosis creates the right environment for planning for future treatments and making an advance directive. Once the "shared silence" has been broken, effective collaboration in advance medical planning can begin.

Educating the Community

Although the PSDA requirements go into effect at the time of admission to a health care facility or managed care program, this is usually not the best time to discuss end-of-life issues. The day of admission is highly stressful for patients, and it is unlikely that they will hear or fully comprehend information given by a clerk with whom they have had no prior relationship. Increasing public awareness and knowledge about advance directives before admission is not just a provision of the PSDA, it is at the very heart of the legislation.[26]

Information about advance directives, living wills, and durable powers of attorney is often transmitted through brochures and newspaper or magazine articles or by lectures and discussion panels. Videotaped presentations (see Appendix D) are also effective in focusing attention on actual or fictional cases that illustrate the benefit of having a living will and/or a durable power of attorney. But an even more compelling way to reach people about these issues is through theater. "Staged readings" of plays such as those presented in this volume provide an excellent entrée to discussion. These discussions can be enhanced by including clergy, social workers, doctors, nurses, and medical personnel and students, some of whom will enjoy playing a role in the readings. As a result of the PSDA, many health care agencies and institutions now have speakers' bureaus that can supply the names of individuals who are prepared to lead community education sessions. Appendix D provides several sources for educational and audio-visual materials that can supplement these presentations.

Churches and synagogues, social service organizations, nursing and retirement homes, schools and universities are appropriate target sites for this community education effort. Most of these organizations already have a vested interest in public education, and their curricula and meeting schedules offer opportunities for presentations on advance planning.

Undertaking a Medical Theater Program

We at Pennsylvania State University's Hershey Medical Center decided to mount a medical theater program as a part of our community outreach. We were aware of the widespread use of drama in various forms as an educational device in medical humanities programs;[27] in particular we knew of Nancy King's innovative and highly successful community outreach program in readers' theater at the University of North Carolina Medical School at Chapel Hill.

We decided to hold a statewide competition — which we called the Pennsylvania Medical Drama Contest — for one-act plays on issues that patients, their families, and their physicians faced at the end of life. Our announcement indicated that suitable plays would be performed as staged readings, with discussions between cast and audience following each performance. Since our cast would be made up of medical students, faculty, and staff at Hershey Medical Center, our after-play discussions would be an opportunity not just to educate the community about advance directives but also to create an open dialogue between health-care providers and the people they serve about the many deep and troubling problems associated with death and dying, especially in a hospital setting. We were able to offer cash awards through the generosity of the Doctors Kienle Center for Humanistic Medicine at the Pennsylvania State University's College of Medicine.

The three scripts reprinted here are the winning plays from that contest. All three plays were performed throughout the year both at the Medical Center and for community audiences. Our program proved so successful that we plan to repeat it, focusing on a different medical issue each year.

The success of our medical theater program encouraged us to think that others might be interested in performing the plays reprinted here, or might even want to mount a program of their own. Toward this purpose, it may be helpful to describe our methods — and our mistakes — in some detail.

Our decision to use original scripts rather than existing plays proved a good one. Soliciting scripts on end-of-life issues from the general public served our mission of community outreach; moreover, it allowed us to secure plays that we could perform as staged readings and that would be short enough to permit a discussion to follow the reading. Ease of performance was and remains crucial to our project: not only do we lack the technical apparatus and staff necessary for an elaborate production, but also, in order to involve busy physicians and medical students, we have to keep rehearsal and even performance time to a minimum. What we wanted — and what we received — were plays short enough to be quickly prepared, simple enough to be performed anywhere, and provocative enough to create excited and exciting discussion.

We were pleased to find a surprising number of talented and ambitious playwrights in the community; we were also pleased in finding a similar vein of acting talent concealed within our medical school. Open auditions provided us with actors to cast all three plays. Double-casting minor roles permitted wider participation by medical faculty as well as by medical students whose clerkships often took them away from Hershey. We found that a capable director could maximize the little rehearsal time we had as well as bring out the best in our amateur actors. One long rehearsal — plus some additional time for work with individual characters — proved sufficient for each play. A further benefit of our medical theater program was the subtle lessons it afforded those who acted in our plays. In performing their parts, medical students and health care providers had to imagine themselves as patients or their families; the healers became the dying.

Of course we needed to attract audiences as well as actors. Our first performance was poorly attended, and it taught us two lessons: try to fit readings into a pre-existing group or class, and make sure each performance is well publicized. We had good attendance and lively participation for almost all our later readings and discussions because we performed for established groups at local churches or for particular classes at nearby colleges. We were helped in finding suitable audiences by our local pastors' association and the medical school's public relations personnel; next year we plan to enlist the help of the hospital's patient advocate to reach community organizations such as library programs and various citizen interest groups.

For reasons that will now be clear, our actual productions remained very simple. All we required were music stands for actors' scripts, and we tried to use swivel-chairs or stools rather than chairs whenever possible. Each play called for a few simple props — a rose, a couple of posters, a novel, and a baseball cap, for example — but these were kept to a minimum. It proved helpful for directors to visit performance sites beforehand whenever possible to make sure the acting area was adequate and visible, to assess the lighting, and to determine whether actors would need microphones. We learned by experience that performances for the elderly present special problems of audibility: each actor requires a microphone, and even then, actors need to "project" and make sure they can be heard.

A reading performance differs from a radio play on the one hand and from full production on the other. Actors read from their scripts, but their acting is not purely vocal. They often turn to look at the character whom they are addressing, and eye contact and facial expression are important to actors and audiences alike. Given the variety of acting space and the limits of rehearsal time, blocking was simple or nonexistent. Though minor characters would at times enter or leave the acting space, the principal actors remained seated, often indicating an entrance or exit simply by facing the audience or turning away. Gestures and physical contact between actors were used sparingly and thus became very powerful. Indeed, these stripped-down performances proved, once again, that in the theater less is often more: our audiences were moved often to laughter and sometimes close to tears.

We used the same format in presenting all three plays. After the actors took their places on stage, the discussion leader welcomed the audience and introduced the topic the play would address. We usually began by asking whether anyone in the audience remembered Nancy Cruzan (usually one or two would). We then used that famous case (discussed above) to lead into an explanation of the Patient Self-Determination Act and advance directives. We brought copies of a model advance directive used by Hershey Medical Center that we distributed after the play. The leader also encouraged the audience to be ready for the discussion to follow, suggesting that they be thinking of questions or problems they might wish to raise. As a transition from this introduction to the play itself, the leader described how a reading performance differs from either a full production or a simple reading of the script, and invited the audience to use their imagination to picture the stage setting, costumes, and action. At this point the leader paused, stepped back, and began to read—very slowly—the initial stage directions written by the playwright. With the audience's attention thus focused on the stage and actors—their collective imagination creating the illusion that is the essence of theatrical reality—the staged reading began.

The reason for this detailed account of the way the plays were created and produced is that what was done at Hershey can be done at other medical schools and hospitals—with variations and, no doubt, with improvements. But the present volume of plays and discussion is not addressed only to medical personnel or medical humanities faculty; we are convinced that our medical theater project can be adapted to any group or organization mounting educational programs on end-of-life issues. Interested persons or groups who feel they need more information to perform one of our plays or mount a medical theater project are invited to contact any of the editors of this volume at the Department of Humanities, the Milton S. Hershey Medical Center, The Pennsylvania State College of Medicine, Hershey, Pennsylvania.

Conclusion

It is no accident that drama — not only films and videotapes but exercises in role-playing and scenic improvisations — is proving an increasingly popular and useful tool for teachers of medical humanities. But this coming together of medicine and drama reflects a much wider cultural phenomenon. Increasingly we see commercial plays and films on medical themes like death and dying. Popular television series are located in hospitals and peopled with doctors, nurses, and their patients, while educational television regularly features documentaries on such topics as healing, alternative medicine, the treatment of mental illness, and the recent evolution of hospices and support groups. The present crisis in health care and the fierce debate on how it can best be delivered and financed is bringing medicine into the headlines of newspapers and the forefront of public consciousness. But beyond all these factors there is the fact that medicine is inherently and essentially dramatic. Death and dying have been central to drama from antiquity: a play that deals with such a subject speaks to all who must confront the death of patients, the death of loved ones, and their own eventual death — it speaks, in other words, to everyone.

It is obvious, then, that the plays that follow address themselves to a much wider audience than educators or medical professionals. They situate the important but narrow topic of advance medical directives and health care proxies in the larger context of end-of-life issues: their real theme, then, is dying and death. Though they are brief — no more than half an hour acting time — each play, in its own way, makes real for us some aspect of the difficulties surrounding the end of life in an era of high-tech medicine. We have already mentioned the shared silence that surrounds dying and death in our society, and it was one purpose of the discussions that followed our plays to break that silence, to open dialogue between a medical cast and a lay audience on topics that seem, for different reasons, forbidding or even forbidden to both. And, as is the way with drama, these topics were articulated, not in abstractions and slogans like "the right to die" or "the sacredness of life," but in concrete and specific human situations involving individual suffering and choice — just as they arise for us in reality. To experience these plays is to confront issues with which our society and each of us must come to terms. And we can experience them in reading as well as in performance. For good theater always involves a necessary act of the imagination. It is our hope that every reader of these plays — plays that are meant for everyone — will picture their performance in the theater of the mind, which may be the best theater of all. In this way the silence will be broken, and the dialogue will go on.

Notes

1. *Cruzan v. Director, Missouri Dept. of Health*, 110 S. Ct. 2841 (1990).
2. *Schloendorff v. New York Hospital*, 211 N.Y. 125, 105 N.E. 92, 93 (1914).
3. *Olmstead v. United States*, 277 U.S. 438, 478 (1928) (dissenting opinion).
4. Jay Katz, *The Silent World of Doctor and Patient* (New York: Free Press, 1984), p. 61.
5. *Natanson v. Kline*, 350 P.2d 1093 (Kan. 1960); *Canterbury v. Spence*, 464 F.2d 772, 784 (D.C. Circ 1972).
6. *In the matter of Quinlan*, 70 N.J. 10, 355 A. 2d 647, cert. denied sub nom., *Garger v. New Jersey*, 429 U.S. 922 (1976).
7. *In the matter of Storar*, 52 N.Y. 2d 363, 420 N.E. 2d 64, cert. denied, 454 U.S. 858 (1981).
8. *Cruzan v. Harmon*, 760 S.W. 2d 408 (Mo. 1988) (en banc).
9. George J. Annas, "Nancy Cruzan and the Right to Die," *New England Journal of Medicine* 323 (1990): 670–73.
10. Larry Gostin and Robert F. Weir, "Life and Death Choices After *Cruzan*: Case Law and Standards of Professional Conduct, *Milbank Quarterly* 69 (1991): 143–72.
11. Omnibus Budget Reconciliation Act of 1990, Pub.L.No 101–508, Sections 4206, 4751, 42, U.S.C., 1395cc, 1396a (West Supp. 1991).
12. Choice in Dying, *Advance Directives and Community Education: A Manual for Institutional Caregivers* (New York: Choice in Dying, March 1992).
13. David John Doukas and Laurence B. McCullough, "The Values History: The Evaluation of the Patient's Values and Advance Directives." *Journal of Family Practice* 32 (1991): 145–53.
14. Susan M. Wolf, "Honoring Broader Directives," in *Practicing the PSDA*, Special Supplement, *Hastings Center Report* 21, 5 (1991): S8–S9.
15. Hastings Center, *Guidelines on the Termination of Life-Sustaining Treatment and the Care of the Dying* (Bloomington: Indiana University Press and Hastings Center, 1987), p. 131.
16. *A Matter of Choice: Planning Ahead for Health Care Decisions,* prepared for use by the Chairman and Ranking Minority Member, Special Committee on Aging, United States Senate; revised by American Association of Retired Persons (Washington, DC: American Association of Retired Persons, 1992). Information in the rest of this section also comes from this document.
17. Elizabeth R. Gamble, Penelope J. McDonald, and Peter R. Lichstein, "Knowledge, Attitudes, and Behavior of Elderly Persons Regarding Living Wills," *Archives of Internal Medicine* 151 (1991): 277–80; Bernard Lo, Gary A. McLeod, and Glenn Saika, "Patient Attitudes to Discussing Life-Sustaining Treatment," *Archives of Internal Medicine* 146 (1986): 1613–15.

18. Linda L. Emanuel, Michael J. Barry, John D. Stoeckle, Lucy M. Ettelson, and Ezekiel J. Emanuel, "Advance Directives for Medical Care — A Case for Greater Use," *New England Journal of Medicine* 324 (1991): 889–95.

19. Kent W. Davidson, Chris Hackler, Delbra R. Caradine, and Ronald S. McCord, "Physicians' Attitudes on Advance Directives," *Journal of the American Medical Association* 262 (1989): 2415–18.

20. Personal communication, Director of Admissions, University Hospitals, M.S. Hershey Medical Center.

21. Gamble et al., "Knowledge, Attitudes, and Behavior"; John La Puma, David Orentlicher, and Robert J. Moss, "Advance Directives on Admission: Clinical Implications and Analysis of the Patient Self-Determination Act of 1990," *Journal of the American Medical Association* 266 (1991): 402–5.

22. Emanuel et al., "Advance Directives."

23. Susan M. Wolf, Philip Boyle, Daniel Callahan, Joseph J. Fins, et al., "Sources of Concern About the Patient Self-Determination Act," *New England Journal of Medicine* 325 (1991): 1666–71.

24. Linda L. Emanuel and Ezekiel J. Emanuel, "The Medical Directive: A New Comprehensive Advance Case Document." *Journal of the American Medical Association* 261 (1989): 3288–93.

25. Katz, *Silent World*, p. 61.

26. Choice in Dying, *Advance Directives*.

27. David H. Flood and Rhonda L. Soricelli, "The Seventh Chair: An Audience Encounter," *Literature and Medicine* 12, 1 (1992): 42–64; William J. Donnelly, "Experiencing The Death of Ivan Ilyich: Narrative Art in the Mainstream of Medical Education," *Pharos* (Spring 1991): 21–28.

Part II

The Plays

Berry L. Barta

Journey Into That Good Night

1992 First Prize Winner, Pennsylvania Medical Drama Contest

About the Author

Berry Barta lives in Indiana, Pennsylvania, with her husband. She was a returning student at Indiana University of Pennsylvania at the time she wrote her play. Barta was raised in rural northeast Nebraska, where she attended primary school in a one-room country schoolhouse. She graduated in a high school class of thirty-three students and went on to the University of Nebraska at Lincoln, which she left in her freshman year. Barta's education continued, though not on a college campus: she held a series of jobs including waitressing, twice serving as a clerk in a hospital emergency room, working as a secretary at two universities, selling cigarettes on street corners in San Francisco, and figuring author royalties at a university press. *Journey Into That Good Night* is the first piece of writing Barta has submitted for competition or publication; partly due to its success, she is at this time at work on another play.

Author's Introduction

My father, Willard Barta, a lifelong farmer, died of heart disease at the age of sixty-six. He'd been ill for many years, so his death was not unexpected. But what was unexpected were the kind of questions he asked toward the end of his life. Had he done enough? Would he have a good death? What would he be remembered for?

In our aging American society there is much interest concerning how to end our lives with dignity, yet discussion is rare and answers are few. Gina Calder's quest for answers and knowledge about the meaning of her life and imminent death in *Journey Into That Good Night* is aided by poetry, immortal poetry written for us all by William Carlos Williams, Alfred, Lord Tennyson, W. H. Auden, William Blake, and Robert Burns. Their genius articulates all that we find too difficult and painful to articulate ourselves.

If poetry can assist us in resolving timeless and universal questions regarding life and death, then hopefully drama will serve the same purpose with societal questions by emphasizing their cultural and immediate character. For instance, are we obliged to take on a special "role" when we are dying? Is the health care profession obliged to go along with that role? And who decides when our role, our life, should end?

Accordingly, Willard Barta's questions about his life and death become Gina Calder's questions. And these concerns are poignant proof that within each corporeal body, belied by the façade of illness, resides a passionate human being longing to be recognized.

So it is with Gina Calder. She is a young but dying college student, struggling with issues of separation from family and community that we demand of someone her age. Yet her illness makes her dependent upon these same institutions, while adding the burden of an unwished-for new community—her health care providers. This paradox of separation versus dependence is resolved by Gina's passionate love of poetry. It is this passion that gives her life and death substance and forces her inherent true nature onto those who care for her.

Willard Barta's true nature, then, was his passionate love of farming. His enthusiasm for the earth and the environment, like Gina Calder's passion for ideas and words, determined the quality of his life and death.

I'll remember my father always on a green John Deere tractor, a red Dekalb seed-corn cap shielding his head, plowing in the springtime, planting corn after the plowing, his sun-squinted eyes on the lookout for crooked corn rows (a sure sign of an uncaring farmer), plowing or planting late into the night, until all that could be heard or seen was the drone of the tractor and the beaming of its headlights far away in the field. He died suddenly in his garden from the exertion of picking sweet peas. I'll always remember that.

The reference to William Carlos Williams's writing "The Red Wheelbarrow" while a young girl was dying comes from X. J. Kennedy, *Literature: An Introduction to Fiction, Poetry, and Drama,* 5th ed. (New York: Harper-Collins, 1991), 532–33, as excerpted from Geri M. Rhodes, "The Paterson

Metaphor in William Carlos Williams's 'Paterson,'" (master's essay, Tufts University, 1965) as told to Rhodes by the director of the Rutherford, New Jersey Public Library. The reference to Williams as Allen Ginsberg's pediatrician and a graduate of the University of Pennsylvania comes from Kennedy, *Literature*, 481.

Journey Into That Good Night

CAST OF CHARACTERS

GINA CALDER: a college student and a hospital patient
THERESA CALDER: Gina's mother
DR. THOMAS: Gina's physician

SETTING

The stage is bare except for a hospital bed center stage. This is the only part of the stage that is lit.

Surrounding the bed is the usual hospital-room furniture: one chair to the left of the bed, another chair to the right, a nightstand with the obligatory sick-bed houseplant on it, and a curtain on the entrance side of the hospital bed. In addition, stacks of books and the personal belongings of a college-age woman are scattered about.

GINA is in the hospital bed; she is young, obviously ill, and resignedly tired. GINA is wearing a hospital gown and a baseball cap. Over her bed is a sign: "I'm Still Alive: Look At Me When You Talk To Me."

THERESA CALDER is a middle-aged mother. She sits in the chair by the nightstand, her purse hanging on one side of the chair. On the floor is her tote bag full of romance novels, magazines, and newspapers; a Danielle Steel novel is also on the floor by her chair. She is dressed in a blouse, slacks, and walking tennis shoes.

SCENE ONE

THERESA: (*on her hands and knees on the floor using colored markers to write on a large piece of white paper*) Gina, why are we doing this again? Isn't that sign we made last week for over your bed good enough? Why another one?
GINA: Come on Mom, from now on we're going to make a new sign each

day. That way everyone in this stupid hospital will know that I'm alive and that I'm going to live forever.

THERESA: But I don't even know what this one means.

GINA: If you wouldn't read all that romance junk you might understand the significance of this new sign. There are great romances in the classics, you know. You should be reading Shakespeare and Sophocles instead of all that Danielle Steel junk.

THERESA: (*sitting back on her heels*) Don't belittle what I do with my time just because you're in college. I'll read whatever I damn well feel like reading. Listen, I would've loved to have been able to go to college.

GINA: Jesus Mom, was that a lecture?

THERESA: You lectured me, so there. And you're sick, Gina, so you shouldn't be taking the Lord's name in vain like that.

GINA: What, swearing's made me sick?

THERESA: (*getting up and sitting on the chair*) You're sick Gina, really sick this time, so you shouldn't upset yourself and everyone who's trying to help you. We all care about you so much and then you put up these signs and swear.

GINA: (*talking into space*) Yeah, you all want me to be Dylan Thomas's patsy and go gentle into that good night shit. Well, I won't! Like the sign above my bed says, "I'm Still Alive: Look At Me When You Talk To Me."

THERESA: Of course you're alive. Don't get all silly now.

GINA: And tomorrow you're all going to get the new sign: "I'm Antigone; I'll Never Die, But You Will." (*Turns to her mother.*) Oh, I don't mean you Mom, I don't mean to hurt you. It's just that I'm so incredibly tired this time.

THERESA: Then who do you want to hurt, Gina? All this outrageous stuff is just hurting you.

GINA: It's my doctor and those nurses and all those techs. They come to see me but they only talk to my chart. My chart has become the patient. "Gina, how are you doing today?" they ask my chart. To my chart, not even me! They won't even look at me.

THERESA: These are busy people, Gina. They do what they've got to do so they can get through the day. And you're so nasty to them — that's why they only talk to your chart. I notice these things too Gina, not just you. You've got to learn to accept them.

GINA: I'll never accept being like them. You know, in anthropology we studied some group of people — God, that class was just last year and I've forgotten so much. Do you think that when I get better I'll have lost my memory of everything I learned in school?

THERESA: Gina, why dwell on college so much?

GINA: No, no, it's all coming back to me now. Anyway, the people in this one culture believe that the dead never leave us physically — get it? Their *bodies* remain behind. The only way you can tell if someone's dead is to touch them. If they're cold, they're dead, even though they still talk and walk. I touch all these hospital people and most of them feel cold. They're fucking dead, Mom!

THERESA: That's enough Gina! Stop it — just stop it! Stop swearing! We've got to stop playing these games and no more signs. Two is enough! (*Starts fumbling in her tote bag.*)

GINA: Two *isn't* enough because I've got to somehow let these zombies know that I'm going to be around for a long time.

THERESA: (*pulls papers out of tote bag*) But we've got to start talking about these — this living will thing — and you've got to start letting your grand-parents and your cousins — your *family* — come and visit you. I believe you're going to live forever too, but we have important things to talk about, and you have to stop shutting us all out.

GINA: There's no need to talk about anything because I can just feel it that I'm going to get stronger and be able to read stuff and write poetry again.

THERESA: So what do signs and the guessing games have to do about anything? What are you trying to prove by all this?

GINA: (*tiredly*) Do you know how I came up with this sign idea? (THERESA *resignedly shakes her head no.*) From here in the hospital — from the techs. They told me this story the last time I was in. Some young woman is brought here from a car accident. The techs said she'd hit the rearview mirror with her face — took off her nose and now she's blind, too. Well, the nurses put a sign over her bed and didn't tell her. It said, "I am blind. Please identify yourself when you enter the room." The blind woman found out about it and ripped it down. *That's* how I came up with this idea. (*Bitterly.*) I bet the blind woman's doctor told the nurses to put that sign up.

THERESA: Gina, Dr. Thomas is good to you. He understands you be-cause he's young, too. Look how he puts up with your guessing games. And your nurses are wonderful, Gina. They're very good to you. You're just being unfair again.

GINA: But they're not sick — *I'm* sick and I *hate* them. They have their educations and they're getting to do what they were trained to do. No matter what happens to them now, they've done something that matters. People will remember them.

THERESA: Is that what this is all about? You won't see your family because you think they won't remember you? Gina, they're begging to come and see you.

GINA: But I haven't done anything important yet. I'm just wasting time here that could be used to be in school. But I'm going to get better. Always before I've gotten better, I'm just more tired this time. Like, this time I feel like a dried-up leaf, all brittle and ready to float away.

THERESA: (*plaintively*) Gina, baby, we've got to talk.

GINA: But I don't want to talk about it.

THERESA: But Gina, there are things I have to know. (*Picks up papers again and begins to read from them.*) "Would you ever want drugs and electric shock to keep your heart beating? Would you want to breathe on a machine? Would you . . ."

GINA: I'm going to live forever, Mom. Why are you doing this to me?

THERESA: Because I'm a mother and I know about these things. Let me help you with this. This is something I can help you with, to make it good, for you and the family.

GINA: It won't be good until I've done something lasting, so just get out of here if you don't want to help me get better. Just leave then.

THERESA: (*almost tearfully*) Gina, this isn't easy on me, talking to my baby about this, but I've got to know. You've always been so particular — everything has to be just so — your clothes, the books you read, the way you plan things out. You'd be mad at me if things weren't just right.

DR. THOMAS: (*Enters room while thumbing through a chart. He doesn't look up as he talks.*) Hi Gina, Mrs. Calder, can I come in?

GINA: No!

DR. THOMAS: (*Now he looks up from the chart.*) How are you, Mrs. Calder?

THERESA: (*looking away and attempting to regain her composure*) We're just fine today.

GINA: Hey Thomas: "Are you moved by truth which comes from suffering?"

THERESA: Gina, do we have to play the game each and every day?

DR. THOMAS: Hmmm. (*pauses — ponders — looks at the "Antigone" sign*) Sophocles?

GINA: (*disgustedly*) Not Sophocles — Shakespeare — *King Lear.*

DR. THOMAS: So you have another amusing sign to torture us with and a reference to Antigone too. I'm sure I'm going to hear hospital rumors about a patient of mine insisting on calling herself "Antigone" (*pronounced Anti-GONE*).

GINA: That's how I pronounced it the first time I read it. I adore "Antigone."

DR. THOMAS: (*pulls a paperback book of poetry out of his pocket and sits down*) Well, you've got me reading lots of poetry lately. (*Waves the book.*) My wife's from college lit. I started reading William Carlos Williams because she tells me he was a physician, which amazes me because how did he find the time to write? Anyway, since I know you regard us Docs so highly (*opens book and thumbs through it*), here goes — Dr. William Carlos Williams — "The Red Wheelbarrow."

> so much depends
> upon
>
> a red wheel
> barrow
>
> glazed with rain
> water
>
> beside the white
> chickens

GINA: You haven't changed my opinion of "you Docs" one bit because of that poem.

THERESA: Oh Gina!

GINA: I've had college lit too, so I know about his being a doctor, and he wrote that poem while one of his patients, some young girl, was dying. Your *Dr.* Williams was daydreaming out of a window and writing a poem about a wheelbarrow while someone in the same room was dying.

DR. THOMAS: Is that true?

GINA: Yes!

DR. THOMAS: I'm sorry, but I honestly wasn't aware of that story. I only liked the poem because it's seemingly simple and because I find it amazing that an M.D. could translate his training into poetry. It's all there like a diagnosis — small and self-contained.

GINA: In my English literary analysis class — we called it anal lit (THOMAS *smiles and* THERESA *looks perplexed*) — there was a dumb poem by Tennyson called "The Eagle." I thought the poem was about an eagle gazing down from a mountain, a simple poem, like your wheelbarrow, small and self-contained, but my prof said I was wrong: it was about a king. Well, she was wrong too because it's about doctors. (*Waves toward a large text.*) Mom, it's in that big text someplace. Will you find it and read it? (*Complainingly to* THOMAS.) I still can't read anything because my vision's so blurry.

THERESA: (*thumbs through the text and stops to read*) Okay now, Alfred, Lord Tennyson, "The Eagle." (GINA *mouths the words as* THERESA *reads.*)

> He clasps the crag with crooked hands;
> Close to the sun in lonely lands,
> Ringed with the azure world, he stands.
>
> The wrinkled sea beneath him crawls;
> He watches from his mountain walls,
> And like a thunderbolt he falls.

GINA: An insulting poem in exchange for an insulting poem, Doctor. This one was written about you because it's about arrogance.

THERESA: Gina, stop this! Be nice to your doctor. (*To* THOMAS.) I can't believe she's acting this way.

DR. THOMAS: No, no! (*Laughing.*) Listen, I look forward to learning something new from Gina whenever I come to see her. I really do.

THERESA: (*reluctantly*) Well, okay then, but Dr. Thomas, I need to ask you a favor. Gina should be helping me with these forms. We should be talking about all this stuff, but she won't. She won't even let anyone from her family visit. Her own grandparents, she won't let them come — not one of her relatives. Won't you talk to her about this?

DR. THOMAS: (*turning toward* GINA) Why won't you let your family visit?

GINA: I can't stand to be around people anymore. I'm not myself now.

DR. THOMAS: How about the counselor I've talked to you about, do you think you could talk to her now?

GINA: No. I don't want to talk about this. (*Turns away.*)

DR. THOMAS: (*sighs*) We've worked hard to get you more physically comfortable, but now we have to worry about your mental comfort. We'll be continuing the same treatment plan, but tomorrow when I visit, we'll discuss a strategy for you to cope better with this part of your illness. Think about it. (*Starts to leave.*) Good day Gina, Mrs. Calder.

THERESA: Thank you, Dr. Thomas.

SCENE TWO

(The setting is the same except for stage right, where there is a hospital waiting room-like area with a chair, an end table, and a lamp. This part of the stage is dark for now. GINA *is wearing a different baseball cap, and her new "Antigone" sign is up.)*

GINA: Read that line again.

THERESA: Gina, do I have to? I don't even understand what kind of poem this is.

GINA: I wouldn't brag.

THERESA: Thank God you don't have me read you this stuff when your father's here. What would he think having to listen to a poem about butts, or that one about a woman having sex with a bird — what was her name?

GINA: Leda, Mom, and it wasn't a bird, it was Zeus in the form of a swan.

THERESA: Oh, excuse me, a swan isn't a bird? It would kill your father to know that this is what he pays all that tuition for. What kind of English major will poetry like this make you?

GINA: Listen, I thought you'd like this poem because it's about ordinary things. *(Conspiratorially.)* But more important than that Mom, who is the poem by, and what significance does it have for *our* Dr. Thomas?

THERESA: Let's see, William Carlos Williams. Hmmm. Oh, I get it. Yes, that *Dr.* Williams you two were talking about yesterday. I get it.

GINA: If Thomas has been doing his homework, he'll be able to identify this poem.

THERESA: He is such a nice doctor, Gina. You should have more respect for him and not waste his time with these games.

GINA: He's a stupid man who knows nothing. He can't make me well again and he doesn't even know poetry.

DR. THOMAS: *(Enters room thumbing through a chart. He doesn't look up as he talks.)* Hi Gina, Mrs. Calder, can I come in?

GINA: *(turns away)* No.

DR. THOMAS: How are you Mrs. Calder?

THERESA: We're just fine today but hoping you didn't forget about that talk you said you'd have with us.

GINA: *(speaks over her shoulder)* Hey Thomas: Oh shit, I can't remember it. Read it Mom, will you? *(Turns toward* THOMAS *and her mother.)*

THERESA: Oh yes, now remember, Dr. Thomas, the name of the poem and the author. *(*GINA *rolls her eyes.)*

> Kicking and rolling about
> the Fair Grounds, swinging their butts, those
> shanks must be sound to bear up under such
> rollicking measures . . .

DR. THOMAS: At last, I know one. William Carlos Williams, "The Dance." (THERESA *claps*.) (THOMAS *to* GINA) He attended Penn, you know.

GINA: (*mimicking* THOMAS) And he was Allen Ginsberg's baby doctor, *you know*.

DR. THOMAS: Really? Is that true?

GINA: (*still mimicking*) Really?

DR. THOMAS: Now Mrs. Calder, if you don't mind, I'd like to talk to Gina. Alone.

THERESA: (*surprised*) Oh, of course, Dr. Thomas. But please get her to let her family visit. And please mention this living will stuff. (*Fumbles in her tote bag and hands him papers.*) Please?

DR. THOMAS: We'll see.

(THERESA *leaves the room for the sitting area on the right part of the stage, which is now lit with a spotlight. She sits down and stares into space. Later, she reads her Steel novel.*)

(*In the meantime,* DR. THOMAS *sits down by* GINA *opposite from where* THERESA *usually sits.*)

GINA: Well, are you here to tell me that I'll once again be swinging my butt at the fairgrounds? If you can't tell me that, then leave.

DR. THOMAS: No, that's not why I'm here. I'm here to find out why you won't let the people who love you be close to you. Why not let them visit?

GINA: I told you, because I'm not myself.

DR. THOMAS: But you are. You're not only poetic, you're a poetess. Can't you be that way with your family?

GINA: And what if they're not interested?

DR. THOMAS: Your mother's not that interested in poetry, but she reads and discusses it with you, even when she doesn't understand it, because she loves you.

GINA: But they're my family, they're not my mother. A mother is different.

DR. THOMAS: Well, you've sold me. You've got me reading this stuff in the most illogical spare moments. I was never interested in poetry until I had the privilege of being ridiculed by you.

GINA: (*cynically*) I'm so pleased that you get to read poetry because I can barely see to read anymore. How can I be poetic if I can't even read the stuff, and how can I be a poet if I can't see to write?

DR. THOMAS: Let your family read and write for you. Poetry is your karma, no matter how you absorb or express it.

GINA: And it's my karma to get better, just like I always have before, so there's no need for anyone to have to help me or come and visit me.

DR. THOMAS: Okay, let's change the subject then. What's your favorite poem lately, or some phrasing that stays with you right now?

GINA: Do you really want to know?

DR. THOMAS: Yes. You started me on this poetry quest, so you'll just have to put up with my picking your brain.

GINA: Well, there's one poem. I can only remember a small part of it though. It's from "Musée des Beaux Arts" by Auden.

DR. THOMAS: So, recite.

GINA: So, I will. (*Pause.*)

> About suffering they were never wrong,
> The Old Masters: how well they understood
> Its human position; how it takes place
> While someone else is eating or opening a window or just walking
>   dully along.

DR. THOMAS: What's the context?

GINA: It's about a painting of Brueghel's that shows Icarus falling into the sea and drowning while everyone on shore goes about doing their own stuff.

DR. THOMAS: Hmmm, that's quite poignant. "Suffering while" — what's the rest?

GINA: " . . . someone is eating or opening a window or just walking along." (*Pause.*) I can't get that stanza out of my mind. (*Pause.*) And how about you? Should I hold my breath or have you read something that moves you?

DR. THOMAS: I have. (*Long pause.*) William Blake's "The Sick Rose." (GINA *looks startled;* THOMAS *pauses again.*) Should I read it?

GINA: (*defeatedly*) I don't care.

DR. THOMAS: (*Pulls out his paperback, thumbs through it, and stops. He recites the poem gently and softly.*)

O Rose, thou art sick!
The invisible worm
That flies in the night,
In the howling storm,

Has found out thy bed
Of crimson joy,
And his dark secret love
Does thy life destroy.

(*Another pause, then, apologetically*) I guess it's the nature of my profession that draws my attention to a poem like this.

GINA: (*crying now*) I know I should be letting you know how I want things to be at the end, and I know that I should let everyone visit me. But how can I end this and still be me? How can I do that?

DR. THOMAS: You keep teaching us about poetry, and we will show you how to end things with dignity and love. We can help you that way.

GINA: (*still crying*) You can't help me die the way I want to die because I haven't left anything lasting—I haven't done anything yet. How can I die and still be remembered for eternity?

DR. THOMAS: We will remember you for the rest of our lives. How could we forget someone like you? Look at all you've taught me.

GINA: Don't patronize me. What could I have possibly taught a doctor?

DR. THOMAS: Well, you've made me more appreciative of language and how people use it to express themselves. I pay more attention now to what my patients tell me, or what they try to tell me.

GINA: Is that enough?

DR. THOMAS: It means a great deal to me.

GINA: I just don't know how to think about these things any more.

DR. THOMAS: Then talk to the counselor. She can help you resolve your feelings about yourself and your family.

GINA: And what if she can't?

DR. THOMAS: Talk to the counselor, Gina.

GINA: (*still crying*) Okay, I'll see your counselor. And you'll promise that you won't remember me just as someone who died young?

DR. THOMAS: (*getting up to go*) I promise.

GINA: And you'll keep reading?

DR. THOMAS: Oh, I'm glad you brought that up. Where in *King Lear* is the line you wanted me to identify?

GINA: Which line?

DR. THOMAS: "Are you moved by truth which comes from suffering?"

GINA: Oh, that. I made it up.

DR. THOMAS: You made it up?

GINA: Yeah, I was tired of the game that day.

DR. THOMAS: My wife and I have read and reread all of *King Lear* just looking for that one line. It's such a magnificent play, you know.

GINA: I know.

SCENE THREE

(The stage is bare except for THERESA *standing middle, stage front, holding one long-stemmed red rose.)*

THERESA: *(long pause)* Gina, I've been reading your poetry — Robert Burns.

> And fare thee weel, my only luve!
>> And fare thee weel awhile!
> And I will come again, my luve
>> Though it were ten thousand mile.

*(*THERESA *pauses again and then places the rose on the stage and exits into the wings.)*

The stage goes to blackness.

The End

Commentary

Berry Barta's *Journey Into That Good Night* succeeds because of its vividly realized characters, its genuinely "dramatic" dialogue, and the way it effectively juxtaposes humor in some scenes with pathos in others. It is the story of a spirited young woman, hospitalized with a terminal illness, who refuses to acknowledge her medical condition. Flaunting a baseball cap, she lashes out angrily and articulately at her mother and the hospital staff — especially her physician, Dr. Thomas. But this same physician finds a way to use the poetry she loves to help her come to terms with her approaching death. Gina's resentment toward her doctor and her resistance to the fact that she is likely to die is in part a function of her age: physicians, particularly pediatricians, who have seen the play recognize a similarity between Gina and many of their young patients, and the play permits these doctors to mourn their "Ginas."

The response of a non-medical audience is somewhat different. It is because she is young, spirited, and intelligent that we allow Gina her partly flirtatious taunting of Dr. Thomas and her refusal to confront the possibility that she might die. And yet many of us — young and old, male and female — can identify with her: we, too, feel the urge to direct the anger that arises as a response to our medical condition onto our doctors — especially when our outlook is poor and it seems unlikely that we will get better. We, too, feel more comfortable denying and fighting our illness than we do accepting it, along with the possibility that we might die. That Gina feels she isn't ready to die because she hasn't yet done anything important makes sense, given her age, but any of us can feel this as we approach our deaths — regardless how old we are. The character of Gina "works" dramatically because we can experience, through her, those feelings that we must often try to control or suppress in our own lives.

Dr. Thomas is effective not simply as a foil for Gina's anger but because of the way he actually tries to help Gina come to terms with her approaching death. He is not angered or hurt by Gina's taunts and insults because he understands their source. She has her agenda, which is to refuse, as long as possible, the ominous knowledge that he brings. His entrance into her hospital room signifies the invasion of her mind by this unwelcome news, and she resists the intrusion: twice he asks her permission to come in and twice she answers, "No." One way of resisting the message is to "kill the messenger," and so she teases and torments him with insults and literary quizzes. But he too has his own agenda, which is to help her come to terms with her feelings about her medical condition. Dr. Thomas's name, of course, invokes the famous Welsh poet Dylan Thomas, from whose "Do Not Go Gentle into That Good Night" the play takes its title.

Dr. Thomas is by no means an ideal doctor: when he enters her room, he looks at Gina's chart, not at her, and she does not fail to remind him of this. But he serves for physicians and non-medical people alike as an effective image because he shows us a physician successfully treating a patient whom he is unable to help medically. The dilemma of the physician who must find a way to care for a patient whom he or she cannot cure is all too familiar to most physicians. Dr. Thomas does not resort to useless procedures and ritual tests — the token gestures of active medical intervention that only prolong a patient's hope and defend the physician from a sense of failure. Instead, he talks to her about poetry. Does he read *King Lear* and William Carlos Williams because Gina has taught him the value of poetry? Yes, and no. Dr. Thomas is sincere in everything he says and does: we feel that he really has learned to admire and even love literature, but at the same time we know that he is using the poetry she loves to help this patient confront the reality of her medical condition. If her passion was for baseball, or for painting, he would use that.

Berry Barta has remarked that she feels Theresa is the play's hero. At first glance this seems surprising. Gina is the central character and the action of the play devolves around her illness; Dr. Thomas plays a crucial role in helping Gina come to terms with the possibility that her illness will end in death and not recovery. But it is Theresa who will feel Gina's loss most keenly; it is Theresa who will go on to find poems (such as the one she reads from Robert Burns) that can help articulate her grief, in the same way that her daughter found poetry to express her own feelings. Parents who are left to lament the death of a child, familial caretakers of the chronically ill, adult children with power of attorney who must determine when their frail and failing parents should no longer be maintained on life-support systems — perhaps these figures, in an age of heroic medicine and patients' rights, have not received the recognition they deserve.

Gina is helped with her feelings first by her doctor and then, we hope, by the counselor she agrees to see. Dr. Thomas's concern for his young patient is tempered by the fact that he has many, many more patients like Gina; moreover, when he takes off his white coat and goes home at the end of a day, to some extent he can put aside the role of the caring and concerned physician. But Theresa is pretty much left to herself to deal with her feelings about a dying child. Does she have other children? Probably. Is her husband a support for her, as well as for Gina? Perhaps, but perhaps not. It is thus appropriate that the play ends with Theresa's grief. Gina is dead and Dr. Thomas has other patients, but Theresa will continue to grieve for Gina for a very long time.

A careful look at the poetry Barta uses will help us appreciate the rich undertones of the play. The heroine of Barta's play is clearly a college English major: the dialogue is full of quotations and literary allusions, and the action in which a young woman comes to terms with death dramatizes the rapprochement of medicine and literature. The play includes overt references to William Carlos Williams's "The Dance" and "The Red Wheel-barrow," W. H. Auden's "Musée des Beaux Arts," William Blake's "The Sick Rose," William Butler Yeats's "Leda and the Swan," Alfred, Lord Tennyson's "The Eagle," Robert Burns's "A Red, Red Rose," Shakespeare's *King Lear,* Sophocles' *Antigone,* and of course Dylan Thomas's "Do Not Go Gentle into That Good Night."

Gina, indeed, does not "go gentle into that good night": she rages against the dark as Dylan Thomas would have her do, and her defiance is complicated and intensified by a Keatsian thirst to achieve immortality through her poems. Her imagination is saturated with the poetry she has read, and some of the passages that haunt her have meanings that resonate beyond their immediate context. Auden's poem, "Musée des Beaux Arts," focuses on a well-known painting by Pieter Brueghel, *The Fall of Icarus,* which takes as its subject the death of the mythological Icarus. Icarus was the son of Daedalus, who made wax wings for himself and his son to escape the prison of King Minos of Crete. Daedalus warns Icarus not to fly too close to the sun, but Icarus, intoxicated with his new-found skill in flying, forgets his father's warning and soars upward as if to reach the heavens. The blazing sun softens the wax with which the wings have been made, and Icarus plunges into the sea. Both the painting and the poem are about the very "ordinary" setting in which this extraordinary event happens, and about how it passes unnoticed.

Williams's poem, "The Dance," is very different. It is about another painting of Brueghel's that depicts a group of peasants singing, dancing, and indulging in the pleasures of drink and sex. The two Brueghel paint-ings — and the two poems they inspire — stand for the alternatives of early youthful death and joyous robust life. Gina knows at some level that she is destined, like Icarus, for an early death, but she also feels the need to soar up into the heavens before that plunge downward. She wants "to do some-thing" before she dies so that she will be remembered.

Gina's identification with the mythological Icarus may be obscure and half-conscious, but her identification with Antigone is overt: she hangs a sign over her bed, "I'm Antigone; I'll Never Die, But You Will." Of course, Antigone does die: indeed, she can be seen as an archetype of a young girl doomed to an early and unfair death—and Gina's sign suggests that at some level she is well aware of the fate she so strenuously denies. Moreover, Antigone's death is heroic: she dies for a principle, in defiance of Creon, her prosaic, earth-bound uncle, who stands for the values of the establishment. Elizabeth Kübler-Ross has proposed that denial and rage are stations on the way to acceptance, and that one of the intermediate stages is bargaining: the dying person "agrees" to die if certain conditions are met. Gina's bargain is clear: she will die if she—like Antigone—can be remembered, and not just by those who love her as family. It is poetry that must make her immortal, and since she cannot write her own, it must be the poetry of others. Hence the key role of Dr. Thomas: he stands for medical science, for all that seems opposed to poetry.

Dr. Thomas is Gina's Creon. Her defiance of the medical establishment in the person of her physician, Dr. Thomas, parallels Antigone's defiance of the political establishment in the person of her uncle, Creon. By taunting and quizzing her doctor, Gina is challenging him to enter her world of literature as she has been forced to enter his world of medicine. This process is marked by the transition from Williams's "The Red Wheelbarrow"—a poem which for Gina marks the physician's detachment from the dying young girl who is his patient—to "The Sick Rose," a poem with obvious relevance to Gina's condition (and a poem in Blake's series, *Songs of Experience*). The actor who plays Dr. Thomas in our performances marks this transition by reading the Williams poem rather stiffly and mechanically and the Blake poem with deep and genuine feeling. The difference in Gina's response to Dr. Thomas's reading of the two poems marks the difference in her acceptance of her condition. The first poem evokes a taunting response: "Your *Dr.* Williams was daydreaming out of a window and writing a poem about a wheelbarrow while someone in the same room was dying," but her response to "The Sick Rose" is to break down and cry. Dr. Thomas compares the Williams poem to a diagnosis, but it is through Blake's rose—itself an age-old type of brief and fading beauty—that he is able to make Gina's diagnosis real to her, moving her from isolating, wilful innocence to the sad but human world of shared experience.

It is after this important scene that *King Lear* is mentioned. Dr. Thomas's admission that he and his wife have been searching through the play for a quotation that Gina actually made up — " Are you moved by truth which comes from suffering?" — never fails to draw laughter from the audience. But the scene ends seriously as Gina agrees with Dr. Thomas that *King Lear* is "such a magnificent play." This is the last literary work they mention; this is their final exchange. In the next scene, Gina is dead. It is surely not accidental that *King Lear* concerns the untimely death of a young woman, Cordelia, and ends with all the characters of the play grouped around her dead body. It beautifully reverses the feeling she has expressed earlier on when she quotes the opening lines of Auden's poem, "Musée des Beaux Arts." Icarus dies but no one notices; Gina, too, senses that she is dying and feels that no one is really paying any attention to her.

Gina demands that "the docs" look at her instead of looking at her chart, and, though both times Dr. Thomas enters he is "thumbing through a chart," we realize that he has come to see and understand Gina, and has found, with patience and insight, the special language that can reach and speak to her. But she has also changed him: she has brought out the innate sensitivity — human as well as literary — that prompts his choice of "The Sick Rose," and we believe that he will go on reading poetry and that he will remember her as more than "someone who died young." How far they have come together is marked by their mutual sense of the magnificence of *King Lear*, where a community of individuals bound by grief and love centers upon another young woman who dies too soon. In Barta's play, this community includes Theresa, the human being who is closest to Gina, but — as an addicted reader of Danielle Steel — furthest from her in educa-tion and taste. What Theresa learns from and through Gina is again evident in the change from her clumsy recitation of Tennyson's "Eagle" to the stanza from Burns with which the play ends. Burns, the poet of common life and "ordinary things," gives Theresa the words she herself could never have found to express her grief and her love. The rose she carries, like the rose in Burns's poem, both recalls and replaces the sick rose of Blake. Diagnosis turns to eulogy: "O my luve's like a red, red rose."

Suggestions for Performance and Discussion

We have begun our performance by reading three of the poems quoted in the play. Gina reads William Carlos Williams's "The Dance," Theresa reads W. H. Auden's "Musée des Beaux Arts," and Dr. Thomas reads Dylan Thomas's "Do Not Go Gentle into That Good Night." Besides providing a "warm-up" for the actors, we found that the transition from the rollicking Williams poem to Thomas's somber verses sets the mood for the play, as well as marking the opposition of comedy and tragedy, humor and pathos, between which it moves so effectively.

When the play begins, the characters are seated with Gina in the middle. Gina and Theresa face the audience; Dr. Thomas faces away from the audience to indicate that he is off-stage. Swivel-chairs or stools enable the actors to turn easily. Music stands allow for greater mobility, though actors can make do with lecterns or reading stands.

PROPS

Two signs, one taped to the wall, the other ready to be fixed over the first sign between scenes one and two; two baseball caps for Gina; a large canvas bag containing a Danielle Steel novel, an anthology of poetry including a copy of Tennyson's "The Eagle," a packet of advance directives (or some substitute), and a long-stemmed rose (real or artificial). Dr. Thomas wears a long white coat, carries a stethoscope, and has a book of poetry in his pocket.

CASTING

The success of this play depends on the ability of Gina and Theresa to display emotion effectively but without sentimentality.

Gina. This play needs a strong "Gina." Look for an actress who can portray Gina's feisty, angry moods but who can also show vulnerability and even break down. It is helpful in auditions to have would-be Ginas read passages involving her insolent retorts to Dr. Thomas as well as the sequence beginning with Dr. Thomas reading "The Sick Rose" and Gina's tearful response. Gina must be portrayed as spunky and feisty, but also as sick. We tried to convey a sense of her physical weakness by having the actress show difficulty in breathing. Her labored respiration increases with stress and in the second scene. And, in fact, according to the physician who played Dr. Thomas, this is a symptom that might well be characteristic of a patient like Gina. To emphasize this aspect of Gina's characterization, we looked for moments when she could express her vulnerability, such as her momentary panic when she thinks she has forgotten everything she learned in college, or her admission of how tired she is (in scene 1, before Dr. Thomas's entrance). Gina capitalized on making eye contact at key moments in the play. She kept this at a minimum when she didn't want to discuss her illness or the possibility of dying, and this strongly accentuated those few times when eye contact was established, such as just after Dr. Thomas read "The Sick Rose."

Theresa. The two actresses who portrayed Theresa in our productions had very different acting styles: one was highly emotional (she played the last scene with tears running down her face), the other much more re-strained. Both were very effective. Theresa is a more complicated character than might appear initially. She has moments when she feels real anger at her daughter, and the actress must be able to read these passages convinc-ingly; at other times her voice softens and must convey the concern and love she feels for Gina; Dr. Thomas she addresses in a polite, placating, almost "smarmy" tone of voice. But Theresa's greatest task is to bring off the very emotional third scene with which the play ends. Our Theresa takes a rose out of her bag, slowly puts it on Gina's reading stand, and then recites the Burns poem. This last scene can be very powerful. Its effectiveness will be heightened if Theresa's recitation of the Burns poem contrasts markedly with her earlier reading, at Gina's request, of Tennyson's "The Eagle." Our Theresa has difficulty with "The Eagle," which she reads with an over-emphasis on the iambic meter; on the other hand she recites (from mem-ory) the Burns poem at the very end of the play beautifully, with great feeling.

Dr. Thomas. Though in some plays a role intended for a male actor can be acted by a woman and vice versa, in this play it seems important for Dr. Thomas to be played by a man, since there is a flirtatious element in Gina's feistiness. Dr. Thomas's attitude toward Gina much of the time is one of amusement at her outrageous behavior; at other times we see him gen-uinely moved by the poetry he has begun to read. Throughout, he must convey a sense of disciplined patience. The crucial speech for Dr. Thomas is his reading of Blake's poem, "The Sick Rose." In some sense this marks the play's turning point, for it is through this poem that he succeeds in making Gina understand that she is going to die; moreover, it is through reading this poem that he brings her to a recognition that she has really touched him and connected with him through poetry. Dr. Thomas looks at Gina as he reads these lines with total seriousness and deep concern, though she does not look at him until he has finished. The effectiveness of Dr. Thomas's reading of "The Sick Rose" will be enhanced if he reads the earlier poem, "The Red Wheelbarrow," quite badly. Our Dr. Thomas read the Williams poem with a pause at the end of each line and a longer, also mechanical pause between stanzas.

STAGING

Actors turn away from the audience, facing to the side, when not on stage. For example, when Theresa's stage directions indicate that she is to leave the room and read her book, the actress turns to the side, takes out her Danielle Steel book, and begins to read.

We indicated scene changes by dimming overhead lights. At the first scene change, Dr. Thomas tapes Gina's new sign onto a back wall and Gina changes her baseball cap. In scene 2, Dr. Thomas should appear to enter in time to overhear Gina's remark, "He's a stupid man who knows nothing." Between scenes 2 and 3, Dr. Thomas and Theresa turn to the side; Gina slowly rises from her chair and slowly walks to the rear of the stage, standing with her back to the audience.

DISCUSSION QUESTIONS — GENERAL

1. How many of you have made out an advance directive? (*Typically, few people will raise their hands.*) It seems striking that surveys teach us that while a great many people indicate that they think advance directives are a good thing, very few people have actually made one out. Does this play suggest reasons why this should be so?

2. How much does Gina really know about her medical condition? Does she really believe that she is going to get better? Several times during the play Gina claims that she is going to "live forever." What does she mean by this?

3. Why does Gina refuse to allow her family to visit her, and why does she differentiate between her mother and the rest of the family in regard to this issue? Observe that Dr. Thomas persists in suggesting that Gina should let her family visit. Why does he do this? What other sources of support might the physician recommend for this, or any patient?

4. Why is Gina so angry at Dr. Thomas?

5. Why does Dr. Thomas put up with the ridicule Gina heaps on him daily? Does his job require this of him? Since it appears that Gina doesn't want to deal with the possibility that she will die, why doesn't Dr. Thomas respect this attitude? Why does he feel he needs to bring her to the point where she can accept death? What clues does she give him in what she says or does that suggest that this acceptance is what she needs?

6. Given what you know of Gina's values and personality, how would she make out an advance directive? (*This is a good time to pass out copies of a model advance directive, if you have not done so beforehand.*) Would she appoint

a health care proxy? Would she add anything to the questions indicated here? (*"Here" refers to the living will portion of the advance directive handed out.*)

7. Elizabeth Kübler-Ross, in her famous book, *On Death and Dying*, describes five stages in the dying or grieving process (denial, anger, bargaining, depression, and acceptance). Does this schema help us better understand Gina? If so, how? Which stages do you find represented in this play? What influences can hinder or enable the patient's progress through these stages?

8. In what way are issues of control important in understanding the play's action? For example, how does Gina identify and express her frustration at her lack of control over her condition? Is Dr. Thomas troubled by the control issue? Why, or why not? As you watch the drama unfold, do you feel this tension between characters' need for control and their actual powerlessness?

QUESTIONS ESPECIALLY APPROPRIATE FOR A MEDICAL AUDIENCE
1. To what extent does Dr. Thomas really love poetry and to what extent is he using poetry as a way to reach Gina? Will he continue to read poetry after she dies?

2. How true are Gina and her mother to your experience of very sick adolescents or young adults and their parents?

3. Can you identify with Dr. Thomas? Why, or why not?

4. The play mentions a counselor who will help Gina with her feelings about death—this might be a social worker or someone from pastoral services who has been trained how best to talk to patients about dying. Whose responsibility is it to help patients come to terms with death? To what extent is the patient's own physician responsible for doing so? Do you find the solution this play suggests—that the physician is partly responsible, but will be helped by others—a good one? Is it feasible?

5. Dr. Thomas is a busy doctor and yet the time he spends with Gina seems well invested. How do we balance the needs of our patients with our workloads? And how do we initially assess those needs?

6. Is there some benefit for the physician as well as the patient in talking about dying?

7. Observe that this play stresses the importance of proceeding at the patient's pace and gently encouraging, never forcing, communication about the issues that Gina so emphatically denies. Can you recall instances when you said the right thing but at the wrong time?

8. If the physician is caring for a dying patient who is unable to talk, what other ways of communication are possible?

9. Examine several models of the physician/patient relationship, discussing the pros and cons of each. Which model describes the relationship between Dr. Thomas and Gina? How does each model facilitate or discourage communication and healing?

Marjorie Ellen Spence

Stars at the Break of Day

1992 Second Prize Winner, Pennsylvania Medical Drama Contest

About the Author

Marjorie Ellen Spence grew up in western Pennsylvania. She attended Millersville University, where she received her B.A. in art, then Franklin and Marshall College, where she completed a second major in drama. Her interest in theater is complemented by a strong social conscience. Thus not only has she acted, directed, and danced in community and college theatrical productions, but she has also worked with Habitat for Humanity to build houses in the United States and Mexico and with a church group to build clinics in Nicaragua, as well as traveling during Cold War times to the former Soviet Union as a citizen ambassador with the Friendship Force. Spence lives in Lancaster, Pennsylvania, where she works as Executive Director of the Theater of the Seventh Sister and serves on the board of directors of Habitat for Humanity. She has two grown children and is also a free-lance artist and writer. At this time she is working on a new play and revising *Stars* for full production.

Author's Introduction

Stars at the Break of Day is a play about a woman coming to grips with her father's long illness in a nursing home and an old friend's impending death.

It was written at the time of my sister's terminal illness. Linda died just after I finished the play. Both my parents had died several years before. My mother's was a sudden death, but my father spent two years in nursing homes, suffering with rapidly increasing dementia. I went to see my father in these homes, and I have lasting impressions of those buildings and the people living within their walls.

The characters in the play have personalities based on people I know, or people I met during my visits to nursing homes. Leroy and Russell have my father's characteristics at different stages of illness. Dorothy is similar to a tiny woman who followed me and talked to me during a nursing home visit, and her "carbon monoxide" conversation is one that I had with my aunt, nearly verbatim.

During one of my visits with my father, I met a relatively young man who was living at the nursing home. He was bright and friendly, and he was in a wheelchair. It was a brief encounter — I was so busy dealing with my father — but I thought about this man often after that day, and wondered why he was there. He became the main character in the play.

Norma Bower was an entirely imagined character until last year. During a search for a home-care nurse for my aunt, a person named Norma Barto appeared for an interview and I was stunned. She was so like Norma, as I had imagined her, and she became the vigorous, thoughtful caretaker of my aunt.

Anna Kochek is symbolic of all the people that we walk past when we go to nursing homes — the ones who are silent. They are the ones we try to push from our consciousness, but who haunt our memories still. They are the ones who cause us to wonder what will become of us when we are old.

Many of us have struggled with decisions regarding treatment of our aging relatives. My father had surgery during his last years. It ensured that he would not die a painful death in an emergency room, but this preventive surgery, performed when my father was unable to make decisions for himself, seemed to escalate his dementia as it prolonged his life. I don't have answers regarding medical treatment of the aged; each case is surely different. My own experience has prompted me to write a medical directive, so that my loved ones will know in advance that I do not wish to have life-prolonging medical treatment if I become incompetent.

Stars at the Break of Day is a play that deals with medical issues at the end of life, but more than anything it is intended to be a play about life and the human spirit. It is about the humble dignity of my mother, my father's gentle sense of humor, and the graceful courage of my sister. It is a play about love.

We tend to think of death in terms of darkness. I have come to believe that we spend our lives traveling toward the light. I think my sister believed that, too. I know she is still there somewhere. We just can't see her anymore.

Stars at the Break of Day

CAST OF CHARACTERS

MICHAEL SAUNDERS, 40: a resident at Country Acres Nursing Home
PAMELA BENNET, 39: a visitor at the nursing home
RUSSELL BENNET, 73: Pamela's father and a resident of the nursing home
ANNA KOCHEK, 80: a resident
LEROY THOMPSON, 70: a resident
NORMA BOWER, 35: a nurse
DOROTHY KERNS, 78: a resident

TIME

An afternoon in March 1990

SETTING

The visitors' lounge of Country Acres Nursing Home. There are comfortable sitting areas in the room. Left of center are two chairs — one a wheelchair — above a TV set. MICHAEL SAUNDERS is seated in the wheelchair, watching a basketball game on television. He is forty and has cancer. He is dressed neatly in casual clothing. He has short hair which is graying. MICHAEL is tall — his legs look too long for the wheelchair — and he is very thin, which makes his features pronounced. He is handsome in spite of his illness. His eyes are tired, but sparkle with his sense of humor. ANNA KOCHEK, a very old woman, sits motionless on the couch at far left. She sits there, staring, through the entire action of the play.

When the play begins, a basketball game can be heard on the TV, with cheering in the background.

ANNOUNCER: It's a 3 point lead with 12 seconds to go. — This will be a great game for Coach McGrath — not only winning the game, but winning at home. — Another 2 for Temple!
MICHAEL: No — No — (*He pushes the volume reduction on his remote control and looks at* ANNA.) Anna, they're losing — (*With dry humor.*) My team is losing. They're the underdogs, Anna. Do you understand what I'm saying? The underdogs are losing. I wanted them to win, Anna.

(*He looks at the television and* ANNA *stares. She plays with a small fold of her skirt, lightly rubbing the fabric between her thumb and forefinger.*)

Anna, you can kiss this game goodbye — 9, 8, 7, 6, — (*He hits the volume on his remote.*)

ANNOUNCER: Five seconds to go in the game — (*cheering*) — Hutchison — a 3 point shot. There's the buzzer! — Too little too late for West Virginia.

(MICHAEL *groans and turns the set down again. The sound is muffled as he continues to watch.*)

(PAMELA BENNETT *enters. She is 39, slender and graceful. Her hair style is soft in appearance; her voice and laughter are deeply pitched and warm; her eyes are bright. She is thoughtful and laughs at herself easily. She is dressed in casual clothing — a long, loose-fitting skirt and flat shoes. She walks to a couch at stage right, plops onto it, picks up a magazine and leafs through it without really seeing it. She is preoccupied. She looks up and recognizes* MICHAEL.)

PAMELA: Michael?

MICHAEL: (*looks — recognizes her*) Hey! Pamela. (*He smiles and turns off the TV.*) I wondered if you might show up one of these days to visit with your Dad.

PAMELA: Michael — I'm sure I haven't seen you since high school.

MICHAEL: (*smiling*) You're right about that. (*Looks at her.*) Life must be good to you. You look wonderful.

PAMELA: (*Seeing him makes her a little nervous.*) Thanks. Sometimes it is. Life, I mean — good to me. (*She looks down for a second and plays with a corner of the magazine — looks up again.*) You are the last person I expected to see today. Is one of your parents . . .

MICHAEL: Pamela — I know I just interrupted, sorry — but why don't you join me? (*He motions toward the chair beside him.*) You're too far away for this conversation.

PAMELA: Oh — (*laughs a little*). Yes. Thank you. I . . . I would like to join you. (*She gets up and walks toward the chair.*) You look good with gray hair — you're thinner — (*Pause.*) Michael, why are you in a wheelchair?

MICHAEL: Transportation to the underworld. (PAMELA *sits in the chair opposite him, not knowing what to say.*) Cancer. I've been fighting like hell. For a while I thought I was winning. I wasn't.

PAMELA: How long — I mean — Do you live here?

MICHAEL: Yeah. For about a month.

PAMELA: (*She looks at him and has questions, but doesn't know what to ask first, or if she should ask. She decides to talk about herself.*) I came home just for a couple of days. Flew into Pittsburgh yesterday. Funny the way I feel at home as soon as I get off the plane and hear people talking. People from western Pennsylvania talk in a distinctive way, don't you think? I think we grew up in a separate culture.

MICHAEL: I always knew I was an alien of some kind.

PAMELA: I'm talking too much. I feel very nervous. I didn't expect to see anyone here. I definitely didn't expect to see you here . . . You see . . . I came here for a specific reason, and I can't tell you what it is.

MICHAEL: You don't have to tell me what it is. Where do you live? What do you do with your days?

PAMELA: If I tell you what it is, I may lose my courage.

MICHAEL: You don't have to tell me. Just tell me about you. I'd say we have some catching up to do—if you have time to stay and talk with me.

PAMELA: Have you seen my Dad, Michael?

MICHAEL: Yes. I see him often, but he doesn't remember me.

PAMELA: He doesn't remember anything. He seems so desperate sometimes. I have to help him. I know what he wants—I know what he would ask if he could. Michael, don't tell anyone I talked with you, okay?

MICHAEL: You look so anxious. Don't worry too much about your Dad. He's cared for here as well as he would be anywhere.

PAMELA: Michael, I came here today to kill my father. And I'm afraid—and you're not supposed to be here.

MICHAEL: Beg pardon?

PAMELA: I don't mean kill him. I mean I came here to help my father die. I came here to help him. I know that's what he wants. I know it. I can see the anguish in his eyes, and he is so confused. . . . Oh, God, I can't believe I told you this. You must not tell anyone that I talked to you. Do you promise?

MICHAEL: Yes.

PAMELA: I've thought it all through — very carefully. I'm going to put him to sleep.

MICHAEL: You're very serious, aren't you?

PAMELA: It's the right thing to do. I decided two weeks ago when the vet told me he'd have to put our dog to sleep. I hesitated. You know what he said? "You don't want her to suffer, do you? It would be cruel to let her suffer." He gave her an injection, and as she lay dying very peacefully in my arms—I thought of my Dad, and the surgery they did to save his—to prolong his life. (*Pause.*) What life? — What kind of life is that to prolong? You've seen him. Do you call that living?

MICHAEL: Not in comparison to the way you live. But, Pamela —

PAMELA: So I made an appointment with my doctor, stayed up all night the night before so I'd look very tired, and I lied. I made up a story about insomnia. I was a good liar — if there is such a thing as a good liar. It's surprising the things you can do when you're determined. Anyway, I have sleeping pills. Right here. (*She taps the pocket of her skirt.*) In a little brown bag.

MICHAEL: Pamela —

PAMELA: I don't want to talk about it anymore. I'm really sorry I said anything at all. You surprised me . . . and I'm feeling anxious. Please tell me about you. Tell me about your life since I last saw you.

MICHAEL: I will. I'll tell you all about my decadent life. But I need to say something first. Why not just give it some more thinking time before you do something that could cause you more pain, not to mention the crime aspect and some very sticky legal issues.

PAMELA: (*speaks more slowly, thoughtfully*) There are many kinds of crimes, not just those for which we may be punished. I think his surgery was a crime. And this place has been a kind of torture for him, Michael. In the beginning — when he first came here — he didn't understand. It was so hard. I had tried to take care of him myself in my home, but he became impossible to control. He was disassembling the house — wiring and all. He was always a good builder, you know. He was just getting it all backwards. He was taking it all apart. Then we tried to hire a live-in nurse to take care of him in his house, and she nearly went out of her mind. He thought she was Mom. God knows what he tried to do to her. (MICHAEL *laughs at this image and Pamela smiles back.*)

(LEROY THOMPSON *enters from the hallway. He is bony and feeble, but gets around on his own. Leroy never smiles but he's a lovable old grouch. He shuffles along looking very unstable.*)

PAMELA: (*notices him and goes to him*) May I help you?

LEROY: What's that? (*He wears a hearing aid, but it doesn't help much.*)

PAMELA: (*louder*) May I help you to sit down?

LEROY: (LEROY *always speaks so that he can be heard.*) Hell no. If I sit down I'll never get back up again.

MICHAEL: Leroy! How are you doin' buddy?

(LEROY *crosses down toward* MICHAEL. PAMELA *stays upstage, leaning on the door frame, watching this.*)

LEROY: I'm doin' fine. Except it's hell gettin' old. It's a great life if you don't weaken.

MICHAEL: (*laughs*) Where have you been? I haven't seen you in a couple of days.

LEROY: (*thinks hard*) Hell, I don't know. Damned if I can remember anything. I'll see a fella and know the face, but I'll be damned if I can remember the name.

MICHAEL: You remember me don't you? — Mike.

LEROY: (*glad for the help, but doesn't let on*) Oh — hell yes.

MICHAEL: Are you going to watch the game with me?

LEROY: Huh?

MICHAEL: (*louder*) Are you going to watch the game with me? — There's another basketball game — this afternoon. (*He points to the TV.*)

LEROY: (*appreciative, but still a grouch*) That'd be awright. Don't suppose you have any beer?

MICHAEL: (*tickled as though he's heard the question before*) No — wish I did!

LEROY: I wish you did too. (*He turns and shuffles away.*)

MICHAEL: I'll tell Norma to come and get you for the game.

LEROY: (*keeps walking — small steps*) Yep. That'd be awright. (*He exits.*)

PAMELA: (*to Michael*) What are you doing here with all these old people?

MICHAEL: They're not so bad. Leroy is my pal, and Anna here — Anna's my girl. (ANNA *stares. She plays with her skirt.*) She doesn't say much, but she enjoys my company. I think she has a crush on me.

PAMELA: I'm not surprised.

(NORMA BOWER *appears in a hallway above the lounge with a cart carrying a pitcher of water, paper cups, pills, and other supplies. She is a nurse — a big woman — overweight and strong looking, as though she could move patients easily and without assistance. She does what she's supposed to do and doesn't give any of these old people much thought. She neither likes nor dislikes them. It's a job.*)

NORMA: (*looking at* PAMELA) You can see your father now.

PAMELA: Thank you.

(NORMA *exits with the cart into a patient's room upstage in the hallway.* PAMELA *takes a deep breath and turns to exit.*)

MICHAEL: Pam? (PAMELA *turns to look at him.*) Don't do anything drastic in the next ten minutes, okay? Can I talk to you first? I'd like to talk with you.
PAMELA: Okay. (*Pause. She looks at him and smiles slightly.*) Remember the gang?
MICHAEL: I sure do.
PAMELA: Funny. (*She moves downstage and leans on a chair.*) I only kept in touch with Karen. We talk — maybe once a year.

(NORMA *comes out of the room upstage, then exits down the hallway.*)

MICHAEL: It's been a long time since I've seen any of them. Lives get separated.
PAMELA: (*nods*) Seemed like forever then, didn't it? As though nothing would ever change. (*They both smile.*)
MICHAEL: We had fun.
PAMELA: (*nods*) We did. Did you marry Annette Richardson?
MICHAEL: (*laughs*) No.
PAMELA: I'm so glad. (MICHAEL *smiles.*)
PAMELA: (*standing*) I'll be back. Will you be here?
MICHAEL: I don't have any plans.
PAMELA: Well — I meant — here in this room.
MICHAEL: (*smiles*) I know. I'll be here.
PAMELA: Okay. (*She turns to exit and then turns back again. She looks at him.*) I'm happy to see you.
MICHAEL: I'm happy to see you. (PAMELA *exits.*)

(NORMA *is entering the lounge with the cart. She pushes it to Anna. She pours a glass of water and then picks up a large card of pills from the cart. It has Anna's name boldly printed across the top. Norma punches out a pill, puts it into Anna's hand, and gives her the water.*)

NORMA: (NORMA *speaks with the assumption that everyone is deaf.*) Okay, Anna. It's time for a pill. Anna — put the pill in your mouth. Half the time I can only get her to swallow it if I get her some pop to drink. I don't have time to get you no Cokes today, Anna. You'll just have to take it with water. You hear me now?

(NORMA *takes the pill out of* ANNA's *hand and puts it into her mouth for her, then lifts the glass to her mouth.* ANNA *swallows.* NORMA *checks a list on the cart, then crosses upstage.*)

MICHAEL: What about me?

NORMA: It's not time.

MICHAEL: It is time, Norma. It's time.

NORMA: I'm sorry. But I told you I can't change nothin' without authorization from the doctor. I can't. Believe me. I'll get in trouble. (*Pause.*) Look—you want me to lose my job? I need this hellish job.

MICHAEL: You called him?

NORMA: I left a message. He'll call.

MICHAEL: I'll call him. I'll find him.

NORMA: Look. I told you. I don't know where he's at. He's not in. It's Saturday. He'll call soon.

MICHAEL: (*pause*) Norma—just give it to me now. He won't care—I'll talk to him. He's not going to make me wait when he knows it's getting worse. Besides—my sister is stopping today. That's the reason I'm in my Sunday best, isn't it Norma? I know she calls ahead so you can get me ready. — She likes to think I'm looking good and doing well. It's easier for her that way. (*Trying to be firm, but looking vulnerable.*) Norma, I want something now. It will be very difficult if the pain gets worse, the way it did this morning. I don't think he'd make me wait if he knew.

NORMA: (*pause, softens slightly*) I'll think about it. Maybe I can catch another doctor or some damn thing. Damn. You know it was a hell of a lot easier around here before you came.

MICHAEL: (*without sarcasm*) Thanks, Norma. (NORMA *exits with the cart.*)

MICHAEL: (*looks at* ANNA) Well, Anna, what do you think? Will she do it?

(PAMELA *enters the hallway with her father, stops, and looks over at* MICHAEL. MICHAEL *doesn't see her.*)

MICHAEL: (*to* ANNA) You look nice and comfortable over there. I'm glad. I'm glad you aren't feeling any pain, Anna. (*Still looking at Anna.*) You're pretty. Did I ever tell you that you're pretty? (PAMELA *is touched by this.*)

(MICHAEL *tries to shift his weight in the chair and exhales audibly with pain.* PAMELA *watches* MICHAEL, *waits for a couple of seconds, then talks to her father and brings him into the room.*)

PAMELA: I think we'll sit in here for a while, Dad.

(RUSSELL BENNETT *is in a chair with wheels that has a tray in front like a high chair. He is hunched over in the chair wearing clothes that look enormous on him. He is emaciated, and his eyes have a glazed look. He is playing with a Rubik's cube. Pamela sits beside him on the arm of a chair, stage right.*)

MICHAEL: (*looking tired*) How is he today?
PAMELA: (*concerned for both her father and* MICHAEL) He doesn't know me — didn't the last time either. (*Pause.*) He was so capable and strong.
MICHAEL: I know.

(NORMA *enters.*)

NORMA: (*to* MICHAEL) I'm going to take you to your room and give you an injection.
MICHAEL: (*looks at her with gratitude*) Sounds good to me.
NORMA: (*as she turns his chair*) Want to stay in your room for a while?
MICHAEL: No. No — I'm coming back here. (*They exit.*)
PAMELA: (*Trying to talk with her father. He is playing with the cube.*) Dad? (*He studies the cube.*) Can you hear me, Dad? You look so thin. I'm going to have to get you some . . . Paul said to tell you Hello — and the kids. You'd hardly recognize them, they're getting so big. They still have the dollhouse you made for them — they collect miniature furniture in it. I don't know what will happen when one of them moves away from home — I guess we'll have to saw it in half. They were talking about you just the other day — about the time you took them fishing. (*She laughs a little.*) That didn't go so well, did it? — Neither of them is much like me when it comes to the outdoors. We had some fun fishing, didn't we? — You and me. (*She gently wraps her hand around his forearm.*) I wonder if you remember anything at all. (*He looks at her.*) Do you know who I am, Dad? It's Pamela — it's me.

(RUSSELL *looks at her, puzzled, and then goes back to playing with his cube.*)

PAMELA: (*heartbroken, rubs his back softly with one hand*) I'm sorry, Dad. — I'm so sorry you had to come here. — But you won't have to live like this anymore. — No more of this.

(NORMA *and* MICHAEL *enter.* NORMA *pushes him back to where she found him and turns to leave.*)

MICHAEL: Norma? (NORMA turns back.) Thanks.

NORMA: Yeah, yeah — you were lucky this time. But don't expect me to take any chances on wreckin' my job. This job drives me nuts sometimes, but it's a job, you know?

MICHAEL: Yes, I know. Thanks. Oh — will you bring Leroy in here at 4:00? We're going to watch the game, if I stay awake. You can join us if you like.

NORMA: When I'm a patient here. That's when I'll have enough time to sit on my backside and watch a basketball game. (*She exits.*)

(RUSSELL *tosses the cube on the floor and starts to take off his sweater.*)

PAMELA: (*pulls the sweater back down*) Don't Dad. It's chilly in here. (*She picks up the cube and hands it to him again.*)

MICHAEL: He doesn't need the pills, Pamela. Don't give him the pills. (PAMELA *looks at Michael.*) I know this has been traumatic for him — and for you. You had to watch him wondering where he was, feeling lost and frightened — you had to listen to him asking to go home when he could still remember home. But his memory is gone. He's living in a world inside his mind now, and I don't think he's suffering. (PAMELA *lowers her head, ready to cry.* MICHAEL *moves his chair toward her.*)

(RUSSELL *starts to sing. It isn't a song, or a tune or words, or anything recognizable. It is a terrible sound, half moaning, with strange syllables.*)

MICHAEL: There, you see — he's fine. He thinks he's Pavarotti. (PAMELA *looks at* RUSSELL, *who lifts his chin and sings very seriously. She smiles. Her father begins to take off the sweater again as he sings. She stands beside him and tries to pull it down. He pulls it up again, singing even louder.*)

PAMELA: Dad.

(RUSSELL *sings louder and pulls the sweater halfway over his head so that one arm is stuck beside his head and his face is covered. He continues to sing through the sweater.*)

PAMELA: (*tries to untangle him*) Dad.

(*She looks at* MICHAEL *and, seeing the look on his face, bursts into laughter and collapses into a chair. Both she and* MICHAEL *laugh,* PAMELA *hysterically.* MICHAEL *holds his abdomen.* RUSSELL *is nearly howling — still through the sweater. There is a lull in the singing.*)

(PAMELA *straightens her face and holds it with her hands.*)

PAMELA: Oh, God — I can't believe I'm laughing. I've never seen him like this, Michael. He's so much worse.

(*She starts to cry as she gets up and untangles her father.* RUSSELL *starts to sing, and* PAMELA *begins to laugh and cry at the same time. She frees him and he stops singing.*)

(MICHAEL *winces with pain.*)

PAMELA: Are you okay? (*Wiping her eyes with a tissue from her pocket.*) What a stupid question. Of course you're not okay. Is it bad?
MICHAEL: Just give me a couple of minutes.
PAMELA: Can I do anything, or get anything?
MICHAEL: (*shakes his head*) I just need a few minutes.

(NORMA *enters.*)

NORMA: Russell, I want you to come with me for a little while. (*To* PAMELA.) I won't be long. Do you want me to bring him back here?
PAMELA: You can take him to his room. I'll see him there.

(NORMA *exits with* RUSSELL, *who is singing again, quietly. Pause.*)

PAMELA: Michael, why are you here? Where is your family?
MICHAEL: Mom and Dad died. I was at my sister's house for a while, after the first surgery.
PAMELA: You're not married?
MICHAEL: I was for a while. It didn't work out. She's in Illinois.
PAMELA: Do you have children?
MICHAEL: No. Do you?
PAMELA: Two girls.
MICHAEL: One marriage?
PAMELA: (*nods*) I met him in college. He was studying to be an engineer. He's in sales.
MICHAEL: (*smiles*) Where do you live?
PAMELA: Virginia — Richmond. Did you stay in Pennsylvania?
MICHAEL: No. After college and Vietnam, I was in Boston. I had a great job — worked for an ad agency.

PAMELA: You were good in art. I remember.

MICHAEL: When I got sick, I took care of myself for a while till I couldn't work, then my sister said I could stay with them. I never thought I'd want to come back here, but it was kind of nice — coming home. Brenda has nice kids. But I think it gave her the creeps having illness in the house. Can't blame her, really. I had more surgery at County Hospital and didn't bounce back after the second round, so they sent me here for post-operative recovery. My sister likes it this way. I think she pays them a lot to keep me here. She has the money. I don't mind. Doesn't matter much where I am at this point. Except — you lose control in a place like this. That's the down side. (*He looks at Anna.*) Isn't that the truth, Anna? — Until it's a full moon, and then we just raise hell, don't we?

(DOROTHY KARNS *enters. She is a tiny old woman who is in wonderful physical condition, but is senile. She walks briskly into the room.*)

MICHAEL: (*smiling at the sight of her*) Oh, no. Dorothy's loose.

DOROTHY: (*She walks to* ANNA, *sits beside her, takes her hand, and begins to talk. She enunciates well.*) It's almost time. It's time to go home. You can come with me. I have new shoes and I'm just about ready. (ANNA *tries to pull her hand away, but Dorothy has a firm hold.*) I have these spots on my hands, you see? (*She shows* ANNA *her other hand.*) They tried to poison me with carbon monoxide. I was living in the other house, and the men came and pumped it into my furnace. They didn't think I knew what they were doing, but I knew.

MICHAEL: (*to* PAMELA) Do me a favor. Rescue Anna. Take Dorothy by the arm, walk her to the central desk, and turn her over to the authorities. She'll come with you. All you have to do is listen.

(DOROTHY *beats her approach by getting up and walking quickly to Pamela. She takes* PAMELA's *hand and walks her to the other side of the room.*)

DOROTHY: Do you see these spots on my hands. It was the carbon monoxide incident. They tried to poison me, but they couldn't do it. It was the furnace, and I heard the noise, and then . . . (*She looks confused.*) I don't remember.

PAMELA: Oh, that's too bad. I'm glad you're all right.

MICHAEL: Better get her to the desk while you have the chance.

PAMELA: Would you like me to take a walk with you?

DOROTHY: I'm ready to go home now. Are you going to take me home?
PAMELA: No, I'm sorry, I can't do that. But I could get you a drink of water. Your mouth seems very dry. Are you thirsty? I'd be glad to get you a glass of water.
DOROTHY: (*very sweetly*) No, thank you. I just had some carbon monoxide.

(PAMELA *swings around toward Michael, and they both have to laugh.* DORO-THY *heads back toward* ANNA, *but* PAMELA *catches her.*)

PAMELA: Dorothy—that's her name, isn't it—Dorothy?
MICHAEL: That's her name.
PAMELA: Dorothy, I would like to go for a walk with you. Will you come with me? Let's go this way.
DOROTHY: (*as they exit*) I'm just about ready. You're my nice friend and you can come with me. (*Her voice fades down the hallway.*) You can come home with me to my nice house. It's time to go home now.
MICHAEL: (*to* ANNA) I know she drives you crazy, but you have to admit she can be humorous. (PAMELA *enters.*) That was fast. Did she break into a run?
PAMELA: A nurse was looking for her. She's cute, isn't she?
MICHAEL: Yes—unless you're feeling very tired and she isn't.
PAMELA: Dad went through a stage like that. He was very confused, but he could still take care of himself in many ways. (*Sits in a chair near* MICHAEL.) Your sister, Brenda—do you see her often? Does she visit with you?
MICHAEL: Sure. She comes to see me at least once a week. Brenda cares, she just has trouble dealing with the messiness of illness. This way she can deny it and if that makes her life easier, it's okay with me.
PAMELA: She sounds like a person who likes to have things in order.
MICHAEL: You've got it—clean, very clean, and in order. In that respect, we have no similarity.
PAMELA: I don't know how anyone could keep things in order with kids around the house.
MICHAEL: With great persistence. Her son, Tim, has a tough time with her, I think. Poor clean little guy. I got a note from him today—want to read it?
PAMELA: Sure. (*She takes the note from Michael and reads aloud.*) "Dear Uncle Mike, Thanks Uncle Mike for my neet dump truk! My Mom said you

wanted to have a pixshur of me all dirty with my new truk. And she said I could even make mud. GEEZ—this could be my best day in the whole world! Love, Tim"

MICHAEL: (*smiles*) He's a good little kid. (*Pause.*) So—are you a full-time Mom?

PAMELA: Not any more. They're teenagers.

MICHAEL: Do you have a job outside of your home?

PAMELA: I'm an actress, sort of. I do community theater. I get paid, but not much. I have another part-time job.

MICHAEL: No kidding. That's nice. You're an actress. What kind of roles do you play?

PAMELA: Well, all kinds of roles—drama and comedy, and, well, the last role I had was the Wicked Witch in *The Wizard of Oz.*

MICHAEL: (*starts laughing*) You don't look like a wicked witch!

PAMELA: Well, I know, but I was green and everything. I didn't really look like myself.

MICHAEL: (*laughs again*) Now that I think about it, your nose and chin are a little longer than they used to be.

PAMELA: (*smiles*) Will you stop! Actually, it was fun. My daughter was in the show, too—she was the good witch.

MICHAEL: A couple of cartoon characters.

PAMELA: Yes. Dumb roles, but fun. It's easy to play cartoon characters—real people get complicated and then you have to think about it. (*They smile and study each other.*)

PAMELA: (*takes a big breath*) God. When you're dying you're supposed to look bad. Only you could look like this. (*He doesn't say anything.*) If we were alone, I'd probably kiss you.

MICHAEL: (*quietly*) GEEZ, this could be my best day in the whole world.

PAMELA: Just because it was the dream of my entire high school life.

MICHAEL: It was?

PAMELA: Yes.

MICHAEL: (*having fun*) Well, then go ahead with it. I won't mind.

PAMELA: And you never looked at me.—I mean, you looked at me, but not the way you looked at Annette.

MICHAEL: I guess it was the blonde hair and blue eyes.

PAMELA: Yes, I know. I was going to bleach my hair but my mother caught me.

MICHAEL: (*smiles*) You were?

PAMELA: I was. (*They smile, then laugh. MICHAEL feels pain. He lowers his head and closes his eyes. He opens them, and looks at her.*)

PAMELA: You're in a lot of pain, aren't you? Most of the time.

MICHAEL: Not for long. I hope.

PAMELA: And here I am making you laugh.

MICHAEL: You can make me laugh anytime. It's been a long time since I really laughed. (*He closes his eyes again.*)

(PAMELA *moves beside him, reaches into her pocket for the pills, and puts the hand with the pills on his lap.*)

PAMELA: (*softly*) Do you want these?

MICHAEL: (*Slowly wraps his hand around hers and the pills. He speaks almost in a whisper.*) Yes. (*Pause.*) Yes, I want these. — But I'm not going to take them. — A month ago I would have. But not after watching Leroy, and Anna, your father, — all of the people who live here. You know, I thought I'd seen all there was of courage during the war. But these people — these old people who look so weak — they're very strong, Pam. It's another kind of courage — a quiet, gentle, abiding courage — against all of the odds.

I can keep Anna company for a while, and be Leroy's buddy for a little while longer. I'll get something more to help me with the pain — and I'll wait with them. (*He laughs a little.*) Would you believe they have dance classes here? When I first came here, I couldn't watch them. Now I watch and I see. I think I'm going to teach a drawing class.

And I'll wait. — I'll wait with them.

(PAMELA *looks at* MICHAEL *with an open, sincere admiration.*)

MICHAEL: But I am going to take these away from you — because you are hellbent to kill someone today!

PAMELA: (*feeling guilty*) I only . . .

MICHAEL: (*puts his fingers against her mouth, stopping her in mid-sentence*) I know. You care. You care so much that you're willing to get yourself into serious trouble to help. You're an angel, Pamela Bennett.

PAMELA: Pamela Bennett. That sounds nice. I haven't heard my real name in years. (*Pause as* MICHAEL *looks at her.*)

MICHAEL: Let me ask you something, Pamela Bennett. Have you ever been outside at daybreak on a clear morning?

PAMELA: I probably have — I don't remember. Why do you ask?

MICHAEL: I like to go outside in the early morning. I have a deal worked out with the night staff — they humor me by unlocking the doors and allowing me to sit out back to watch the sun come up. Before the sun rises, if the sky is clear, you can see stars that still shine in the morning sky. And there are always a few—a handful—that shine longest—that hold their own light until the sun comes up. Then they disappear into the day. They're still up there somewhere, we just can't see them anymore.

PAMELA: Michael—it's so beautiful—the way you think about . . . (*her words get choked.*)

MICHAEL: When I'm gone—when I disappear—when your Dad disappears—will you do something for me? Will you go outside before sunrise sometime, and watch the stars and remember what I said?

PAMELA: Yes.

MICHAEL: These people—these new, gentle, peculiar friends—they're like my stars at the break of day. Do you know what I mean? (PAMELA *nods.*)

MICHAEL: I mean, look at Anna over there. She follows me in here every day just to let me know she's here. And you—must be the brightest thing that has ever come into this place. (*Pause.*) I have appreciated seeing you. Thank you.

(PAMELA *touches his face. It stuns him to feel this kind of touch, and he fights tears. She puts her head in his lap and cries, silently.*)

PAMELA: I am the one who should thank. Oh, Michael, think of what might have happened if I hadn't seen you today. You've helped me so much. I feel better about Dad, and I'm glad he's here where you are.

(MICHAEL *touches her hair. They struggle in silence.*)

MICHAEL: (*with humor*) Do you think it's too soon to tell you that I love you?

PAMELA: (*reaching into her pocket for another tissue*) Too soon? (*Blowing her nose.*) Why didn't you tell me that in eleventh grade?

MICHAEL: (*pause*) Because you were weird in eleventh grade. (*They laugh.*)

PAMELA: I want so much to see you again, Michael. I won't be able to get back here for about a month. Will you be here?

MICHAEL: Maybe. But I don't think so. I . . . I don't think so.

PAMELA: (*struggling*) It's not fair that you're going to die. And it's not fair to find a lost friend only to lose him again.

MICHAEL: I agree. Life can be brutally unfair. But I'm sure not sorry that you found your lost friend, even if only for a brief time.

PAMELA: I'm not sorry either—I'm so glad. (*She holds out her hand.*) Here—I'll throw the pills away. I promise. Guess they weren't so important after all. (*He gives them to her.*) Goodbye. I'll—I'll be thinking about you.
MICHAEL: I'll be thinking about you, too.
PAMELA: I won't forget what you said—anything that you said.
MICHAEL: I won't forget you either.
PAMELA: Goodbye, Michael Saunders. (*They look at each other for a second, and then* PAMELA *turns and begins to walk away. She stops and walks toward him again.*)
PAMELA: I love you, too—I really do love you. (*She walks quickly out of the room.*)

(*Silence as* MICHAEL *sits there, alone with* ANNA. NORMA *enters with* LEROY.)

NORMA: The game is about to start.
MICHAEL: (*loudly, so* LEROY *can hear him*) Okay, Leroy. Are you ready?
LEROY: (*grouch*) Soon as I get lowered into the damned chair. (NORMA *lowers Leroy into the chair.*)
LEROY: (*groans*) It's hell gettin' old. It's a great life if you don't weaken.
MICHAEL: Thanks, Norma.
NORMA: Welcome. I talked with Dr. Cross. He's coming over.
MICHAEL: (*drops his head against the back of the chair*) That's good news.

(NORMA *exits.* MICHAEL *turns on the television—low volume.*)

LEROY: (*looking at the TV*) Don't suppose you have any beer?
MICHAEL: (*looks with great fondness at* LEROY) No—wish I did!
LEROY: I wish you did, too.

(SOUND: Sounds of the game swell slightly and then fade as the lights dim.)

Commentary

In Marjorie Ellen Spence's *Stars at the Break of Day,* Michael and Pamela, old high school friends, meet unexpectedly in the nursing home where Michael is dying of cancer and Pamela's father is confined with extreme mental deterioration. Other characters in this play include Norma, a gruff but kindly nurse, and several nursing home residents: cranky Leroy, catatonic Anna, and garrulous, delusional Dorothy. Spence introduces the issue of euthanasia with Pamela's statement that she intends "to help my father die," though the play concludes with her decision not to carry out that intention. The double plot of filial love and romantic attraction complicates the play and its issues in interesting ways.

The play begins in the nursing home as Michael is watching the end of a basketball game on TV. The team Michael favors is the underdog and it is losing, just as he is losing against cancer: "I thought I was winning," he tells Pamela later on; "I wasn't." But the oldest cliché in sports teaches that how you play the game counts more than winning it, and in any case, a new game is beginning at the end of Spence's play. It is the openness of human possibility that becomes the play's strongest argument for holding out.

At the play's thematic center is Russell, Pamela's father, who is the subject of her literal life-or-death decision. He is playing with a Rubik's cube, and the multi-sided puzzle symbolizes the enigma he represents. Michael is confident that Russell is not suffering, while Pamela is convinced she sees "anguish" in his eyes. But the stage directions tell us only that his eyes have a "glazed look": how can we know who is right? When Russell starts to sing, Michael exclaims triumphantly, "There, you see — he's fine. He thinks he's Pavarotti." But this singing, Spence tells us, is "a terrible sound, half moaning, with strange syllables." As he sings, Russell tries to take off his sweater; Pamela intervenes, pulling it down again. But Russell perseveres, becoming entangled with the sweater halfway over his head, his face covered, still singing loudly. Russell's entanglement with his sweater nicely captures his position in life — caught half in, half out, his face concealed. The event is both comic and tragic, moving Pamela at the same time to laughter and tears.

It is Michael who persuades Pamela not to carry through her intention to help her father die. He does this not so much by what he says as by his example: he is clearly in a good deal of physical pain much of the time, whereas it is evident that her father is not. And one of Pamela's reasons for wanting to kill her father is to spare him further suffering. Michael tells her that he has learned to see "a quiet, gentle, abiding courage" in the nursing home residents, though we sense that this courage is very much a reflection of his own. He has learned to make a home for himself here at Country Acres, where he has been left by a sister uncomfortable around sick people.

The play suggests that Pamela's decision to kill her father may stem from her need to relieve her own, very understandable suffering at watching him deteriorate into senescence and oblivion. But as the double plot unfolds, Pamela finds that relief from suffering comes from Michael, who, in this vista of decay and despite his own suffering and imminent death, stands for life. He is able to give and receive love, which some physician-ethicists maintain to be the criterion of a life that is worth living. Michael interacts with everyone around. He is a pal to cranky old Leroy, flirts with Anna, keeps an eye on Dorothy — moves even the gruff and overworked Norma to a human response to his pain that risks her precious job. In turn, they sustain his courage — and his sense of fun. A month ago, he would have taken Pamela's pills; it is what he sees in these old people that makes him decide to "wait with them": they are his "stars at the break of day." In this sense, then, they give as well as receive.

What at first glance may seem an intrusive element in the play — the romance between Pamela and Michael — is in fact at the heart of its argument. Life as these two experience it is disorderly and full of accidents: their stories show no meaningful pattern. Pamela loved Michael all through high school, but he cared only for Annette Richardson, with her blue eyes and blonde hair, and each of them married someone else. But now — apparently still by accident — life brings them together again. If Michael had decided to end his suffering, he would not be there for Pamela to help her in her moment of decision. And neither of them would have realized whom they really love. It is compulsively neat persons, like Michael's sister, who want to tidy up the disorderly end of life, to impose a shape on its ongoing and unpredictable and often painful messiness. Those like Michael and his young nephew who accept all this may experience — even at the end of life — "my best day in the whole world." The game is not over until it's over, and there is dancing even in the nursing home. So Michael tells Pamela that when he first arrived he couldn't bear to watch the dance classes; "Now I watch and I see." What he sees is precisely what Pamela has been unable to see. Michael thus becomes the voice for these residents of the nursing home, most of whom cannot speak for themselves.

This is one way to interpret *Stars at the Break of Day*. But to see the play only in this way is to render it merely sentimental — a warm and fuzzy tribute to the ethical principle that life in any condition is worth preserving. The play has deeper undertones, and it is these that give it depth and power. In fact the play undercuts its ostensible premise — that the lives of these elderly nursing home residents demonstrate great courage and that their lives are worth preserving, if only for this reason. Three of the four elderly residents in Spence's play are demented in some way. Anna never speaks throughout the play: she is catatonic. Russell has lost much of his mental capacity: he cannot even recognize his daughter. Dorothy is delusional: she thinks people are trying to poison her. Her pathetic lament — "I'm ready to go home now. Are you going to take me home?" — can be interpreted as a request to "go home" in the final sense. That she should ask this of Pamela, who actually intends to kill her father, underscores the ambiguity of her request. In what way, then, do the lives of these people convey a sense of courage?

Under its sentimental exterior, the play poses some hard questions — for those who are willing to consider them. What does Pamela's father really want? Or what would he have wanted, were his mental function still intact? Would he, like Dorothy, ask "to go home now"? We don't know the answer, but it is an important question — one that is central to the current debate on euthanasia and physician-assisted suicide. Pamela feels certain that her father wants her to help him die. Though he can't speak, he communicates this request nonverbally: "I can see the anguish in his eyes," she remarks. Is Pamela responding to something genuinely there, or is she projecting her own suffering onto his experience — seeing in his eyes a reflection of her own anguish? The model for her decision is the occasion, two weeks ago, when the vet "put to sleep" the old family dog: "as she lay dying very peacefully in my arms — I thought of my Dad." But there are important differences between killing a dog and killing a human being. Has Pamela worked through the moral implications — not to mention the possible legal repercussions (which Michael mentions) — of what she is about to do? In *not* raising this tangle of questions directly, the play cleverly manipulates us, the audience, into doing so.

Pamela changes her decision about killing her father at Michael's insistence. Comparing her reasons for this change of mind to her reasons for her original intention can be instructive. It is evident that Pamela has given some thought to the decision to terminate her father's life. In explaining her intention, she uses the word "kill," but makes a careful distinction between murder and helping someone die. She clearly sees herself as "helping" her father by this act. Russell's condition is evidently the result of an earlier surgical procedure—"surgery they did to save his—to prolong his life." In distinguishing between "saving" and "prolonging" life, it seems clear that the criterion Pamela is using is quality of life: "You've seen him," she says to Michael, "Do you call that living?" Moreover her decision to commit an act that she knows is illegal, and thus punishable, is based on a hierarchy of values: "There are many kinds of crimes, not just those for which we may be punished. I think his surgery was a crime." Whether right or wrong, her decision to kill her father is a considered one, based at least in part on principle.

But is there as much consideration given to what her father would want in her *reversal* of this decision? One could argue that Pamela is wrong to change her mind about killing her father—that she has allowed her infatuation with the handsome Michael to come between her and her intent. She even gives the sleeping pills intended for her father to Michael, asking softly "Do you want these?" She does this because she realizes that Michael is suffering a good deal more than her father, and that he may be more in need of an assisted death. Michael does accept the pills, though not for the reason she gives them to him. He does not try to persuade her that euthanasia—whether involuntary (in the case of Russell) or voluntary (in his own case)—is wrong; he tells her only that the lives of the nursing home residents demonstrate courage—"a quiet, gentle, abiding courage"—a lesson he has learned from living among them. And yet Michael's argument about courage really only applies to him: he is the only character suffering physical pain (and the only character, one might argue, even capable of mental pain). The play ends with a budding romance, even though it also ends with a strong sense of farewell. Michael has, to some extent, replaced Russell in her affections, and she permits him to interfere with her plan without ever convincing her that it is wrong. If Pamela does not give any reasons for not killing her father, it is because she has none. Seen in this light, Pamela's "change of heart" is deeply troubling.

This play, so deceptively simple, shows us just how complicated issues surrounding the elderly at the end of life really are. There is no easy answer, though those at extreme positions in the debate on euthanasia might think so. Before we, as a society, will know what stand to take on these issues, we must think deeply and long about them.

Though this play does not center on the subject of advance medical directives—in fact it never mentions them—it may well provide the most convincing proof in all three plays of the need for them. If Russell had made out a living will before his surgery, and if this directive indicated conditions under which he would not want to live, then his present situation at Country Acres Nursing Home might have been avoided; moreover, if he had named his daughter as his health care proxy as well, then Pamela might well have made a decision to terminate life support systems that would have ended his life before the operation that served to prolong it. It is undeniable that this, too, is an act of killing, though ethicists have evolved linguistic distinctions that might imply it is not. But the differences between this and the involuntary euthanasia that she intends are considerable: when death results from enacting an individual's advance medical directive, it conforms to that person's wishes, it bears the stamp of societal consensus, and it is legally sanctioned. It is the difference between the death of a pet and the death of a human being.

Suggestions for Performance and Discussion

In some ways, this seemed the most difficult of the three plays to perform well. We were concerned that youthful medical students playing elderly nursing home residents might turn them into caricatures, and we were anxious about offending older persons — especially nursing home residents — in our audiences. We dealt with this by turning the problem into an educational opportunity. During rehearsals we arranged for the cast to visit a nursing home, talk with the staff and residents, then share impressions and concerns afterward in an informal discussion. All our actors reported a better understanding of the characters they were asked to play as a result of this experience. Some students with strong negative stereotypes of the elderly or of nursing homes were pleasantly surprised by what they saw.

The readings themselves turned out well, though one performance in a nursing home alerted us to problems of audibility that must be expected in acting for an older audience. Afterward we also wondered whether the issue of advance directives was appropriate for a nursing home, where patients would have dealt with it upon admission, and whether the play's concern with euthanasia might not prove troubling. On the other hand, a performance of the play before an audience of Unitarians was quite successful in provoking a lively — even heated — discussion about euthanasia in general and about the possibility of including a request for euthanasia in an advance directive. Genuine dialogue about such important and controversial issues should, in our view, be encouraged, not avoided: it is one of the play's strengths that the moral conflict at its center continues to animate audience discussions when the play itself is done.

SETTING, PROPS, AND COSTUMES

When the play begins the characters are seated, from left to right: Anna, Michael, Pamela, Russell, Leroy. Dorothy and Norma are seated to the side; both walk on to give their lines.

Props (which are optional) include a bag or vial for the pills Pamela brings and a Rubik's cube (a set of keys will do) for Russell. Russell must wear a sweater; Michael is dressed in his "Sunday best." Anna and Dorothy may wish to wear a shawl and/or put their hair back into a bun.

CASTING

This play originally included nine characters. Michael's sister and her eight-year-old son, who come to visit him in the nursing home, were cut from the script at our request because no boy actor was available. In some productions we also cut the part of Dorothy, with the author's permission, to decrease the number of actors required for performance.

The play is easier to cast than it might seem at first. It requires skilled actors for the parts of Michael and Pamela, but other parts can be cast relatively easily.

Michael. The actor playing this role must be sensitive and versatile. Michael's character interacts with all others in this play — with the elderly denizens of the nursing home, for whom he must convincingly show affection or comradeship; with the brusque nurse Norma, whom he must persuade to give him his medication early; and of course with Pamela, with whom his relationship is something between an old friendship and a new romance.

Pamela. It is important to find a Pamela whose acting skills are roughly equal to Michael's and whose voice projects well, even in more intimate exchanges. Moreover, this actress must make us actually like Pamela: we must sympathize with her when, in telling Michael of her intention to kill her father, she describes what has moved her to want to do this.

Norma. This role can be both challenging and instructive. It could be acted several ways: the exact proportion of gruffness to kindliness will vary with the actor or the director's interpretation of the role. Visiting a nursing home to observe some "Normas" would surely enrich the actor's understanding of the part. The role could be played by a woman or a man — a "Norma" or a "Norman."

Russell. This is a non-speaking part, though it involves vocalization and gesture (Russell must "sing" and he must struggle to take off his sweater). It is a role that requires no rehearsal time; on the other hand, it does require tact — Russell's characterization is intended to evoke both pity and amusement. We had physicians play this role, inviting a different person for each performance. This succeeded in involving doctors in the theater project with a minimum expenditure of their time. Because of their experience with the health care needs of the aged, these physicians were invaluable participants in the discussions that followed performance.

Anna. This is another non-speaking part appropriate for an individual who has minimal acting skills but wants to be involved in the theater project. Our Anna visited an area nursing home several times, searching out those residents who best fit her character. She turned out to be superb in this role, staring straight ahead throughout the play with a fixed, vacant, but lovely expression on her face. When Michael turns to Anna and says "Anna's my girl . . . I think she has a crush on me," both actors made us all see her otherworldly beauty.

Leroy. "A lovable old grouch," Leroy is easy to cast and fun to play. In one of our productions he dressed in baggy trousers and a rumpled shirt, allowed his beard to grow, and sported a cane. The audience enjoyed this Leroy: his repeated wish for beer never failed to provoke laughter.

Dorothy. Though a small role, this is a speaking part. Dorothy, like Leroy, needs to be portrayed with sympathy and compassion and not just played for comedy.

DISCUSSION QUESTIONS — GENERAL

Cast members — especially those who are physicians — should be prepared to answer very direct questions about euthanasia. It is important, during the discussion, that differences between executing an advance directive and the various forms of euthanasia be clarified.

1. (*To the audience*): Do you have relatives or friends whom Anna or Russell or Dorothy remind you of?

2. (*To any of the actors, especially those playing Anna and Norma*): Tell us something about how you conceived your part. What or whom did you use as a model?

3. Advance medical directives are not actually mentioned in this play. If any of these characters had advance directives, would it change the action of the play? (*This question could lead into a discussion of occasions and conditions when advance directives are appropriate.*) The play tells us that Russell underwent surgery: how might an advance directive have resulted in a different outcome? Or, to look toward the future, imagine that the play has a second act, in which Russell develops a serious medical condition. How might Pamela best handle possible scenarios? (*Here one might introduce the pos*

sibility of Russell being allowed to die in the nursing home — audience members could be advised how to arrange this.)

4. Pamela comes to the nursing home to kill her father, but changes her mind, at Michael's insistance. Did she make the right decision at the end of the play?

5. Pamela mentions that two weeks ago the vet put her dog to sleep, and that it was this that gave her the idea of killing her father. Is the analogy a good one? Why, or why not? (*Distinctions between the different kinds of euthanasia might be mentioned here.*) Notice that the reason given for putting the dog to sleep is to prevent further suffering. Is Russell suffering? Is he in pain? Is there a difference between suffering and pain?

6. Pamela tries to articulate the moral nature of what she intends to do when she tells Michael that she has come to kill her father — but "kill" as in helping him die, not murdering him. Is there a meaningful distinction here between these two senses of "kill"?

7. What is the dramatic function of the four nursing home residents? Couldn't the action have taken place as a dialogue between Michael and Pamela? What does each of these elderly persons — Russell, Anna, Dorothy, Leroy — bring to the play?

8. Does the portrayal of a nursing home in this play correspond to your experience or that of friends or relatives? What are the benefits and problems of nursing home care? For the residents? For their families? What determines when a loved one should be put in a nursing home?

QUESTIONS ESPECIALLY APPROPRIATE FOR A MEDICAL AUDIENCE

1. Have you cared for patients who you sense do want to die, though they don't actually say so? What makes you feel that this is what they want? How can you find out?

2. Have you cared for patients who ask you to help them die? How should a physician handle such a request?

3. What are some of the reasons behind requests by patients that they be allowed to die or assisted in dying?

4. The concept of "personhood" is a familiar one to medical ethicists. Are Anna, Russell, and Dorothy still "persons"? Why, or why not?

CE McClelland

Time to Go

1992 Honorable Mention, Pennsylvania Medical Drama Contest

About the Author

CE McClelland is a secondary school teacher and playwright. Born and raised in Philadelphia, he attended La Salle University, where he received a B.A. in English-Education, and then Villanova University, where he was awarded an M.A. in Theatre. His plays, which have been produced by regional theaters in several states, have won numerous awards. "Mausoleum Man" in 1988 and "Certain Arrangements" in 1992 took first place in the Comtra Theatre Competition, and "The Score" was a co-winner in the Milwaukee Playwrights Studio Theater Festival of Ten-Minute Plays. Other award-winning plays include "Growin' Pains" and "The Reddition." McClelland and his wife live in Harleysville, Pennsylvania, with a cat named Vivien Leigh. He teaches high school English and a theater course emphasizing playwriting, and directs student plays in the Wissahickon School District in Ambler, Pennsylvania.

Author's Introduction: How *Time to Go* Came to Be

Usually I know what my next play will be about. A theatrical production dealing with "issues that patients, their families, and doctors face at the end of life" was certainly not one on my agenda; therefore, I was taken off guard completely when I received a letter in February 1992 from Dr. Anne Hunsaker Hawkins of the Hershey Medical Center inviting me, as a Pennsylvania playwright, to submit this type of play in a competition.

I found the topic — not to mention the prize money — intriguing, but I had to admit honestly that I didn't know the first thing about the subject. Still, I thought I'd give it a try and called Anne to ask for more information, which she immediately sent in the form of reprints of brochures and articles on advance medical directives. I read the material, thought about it, put it away, and then waited to see whether any of it would be compelling enough to make me want to write.

Nothing happened. Several months passed without my writing a word. Before I knew it, it was late July; the deadline for submissions was three weeks away, and I was scheduled to leave on a European vacation a week before that. This gave me two weeks to write something, if anything.

Once more I took out the material and looked it over. Now one item caught my attention. It was the reprint of a brochure entitled *About Advance Medical Directives,* distributed by Concern for Dying/Society for the Right to Die. The booklet was written in simple language, but what really drew my attention was the illustrative material. I believe it was the cartoon-like nature of each illustration which suggested to me that the approach to such a serious topic as near-death issues need not itself be so serious. After all, if both Thornton Wilder in *Our Town* and Warren Beatty in *Heaven Can Wait* had gotten away with after-death fantasies, why couldn't I get away with a near-death one?

That was it. I'd write a fantasy! The writer's caution, "Write about what you know!" quickly gave way to the writer's more compelling impetus, "What if?" What if a young man had been in a coma for a number of years? What if his parents were divided over the issue of further prolonging his life? What if the doctor could not advise them in coming to a decision? And the biggest "What-ifs" of all: What if the patient knew his coma was irreversible? That life was better on "the other side?" And that he could not communicate this to his parents? What if he found all this out from some otherworldly intermediary assigned to his care? What if, indeed?

In choosing this approach, I found myself experiencing that rare pleasure of having the play somehow write itself. I wrote a first draft and showed it to my wife, Kitty. She, as well as two mutual friends, Louise Herko and Mary Turner, who are nurses, made several suggestions that were incorporated into the final draft. I gave the play the ambiguous title of "Time to Go" and sent it off to Hershey.

Both my European vacation and the subsequent start of a new school year afforded me little time to dwell on the outcome of the contest. Then in mid-September, I received another letter from Anne informing me that my play had placed third in the competition and that it would receive a series of staged readings in and around Hershey by a troupe of medical students and doctors known as the Hershey Medical Theater Group.

I had the opportunity to attend these readings and was impressed by the professional caliber of the performances. I was also personally gratified by the audiences' reactions. The discussions that followed the readings were also very stimulating experiences.

Now that "Time to Go" is being published, I hope it will find a wider audience. More important, I hope the play will enable readers and audiences to focus on this important issue just as I had to when I decided to write about it.

My special thanks to Anne Hawkins for spearheading the performances and publication of "Time to Go," and to the Hershey Medical Theater Group—Rob Biter, Brian Fosnocht, Sherman Hawkins, Lin Wong, Lori Maxfield, Michele Casoli, Jo Ballard, and Theodore Blaisdell—for bringing it to life.

Time to Go

CAST OF CHARACTERS

The PATIENT, mid-30s
The FRIEND, 50-ish
ANOTHER FRIEND, 50-ish
The MOTHER, middle-aged
The FATHER, middle-aged
The DOCTOR, 30-ish

TIME

The present

SETTING

A bare stage with a hospital bed, a night table, and a few chairs. The PATIENT, a man in his middle 30s, lies in a fetal position on the bed. A feeding tube is attached to his stomach. Another man, The FRIEND, sits beside the bed. He is middle-aged with white hair and is wearing a white tuxedo with tails. Paging through a tabloid newspaper, he chuckles occasionally at an item that amuses him.

FRIEND: "ELVIS AND MARILYN SPOTTED IN HONEYMOON HOT TUB" . . . "VICE PRESIDENT IS ALIEN IMPOSTER" . . .

"UFO'S PILOTED BY GUARDIAN ANGELS"—hmm, this one might prove to be interesting.

(Just then ANOTHER FRIEND, *similarly dressed, enters from the right.)*

ANOTHER FRIEND: Hello, Friend!
FRIEND: Hello, Friend!
ANOTHER FRIEND: Still here, I see.
FRIEND: So it seems. How is business with you?
ANOTHER FRIEND: Can't complain. I just completed a crossover. Second one today. I'm on my way to my next case, traffic accident out on the state highway.
FRIEND: Well, good luck.
ANOTHER FRIEND: Thank you, Friend. Well, I'll be seeing you. (AN-OTHER FRIEND *exits.*)
FRIEND: Yes, "in all the old familiar places." Some of us have all the luck. (*Looks at the* PATIENT *on the bed.*)
FRIEND: I have had just about enough of this. (*shaking the* PATIENT) Young man. Young man, wake up. Wake up, I say.

(The PATIENT *uncurls slowly from his fetal position, sits up, and opens his eyes.)*

PATIENT: Who are you?
FRIEND: A friend.
PATIENT: Where am I?
FRIEND: You're in a hospital.
PATIENT: Hospital?
FRIEND: Yes.
PATIENT: What happened?
FRIEND: You were in an accident.
PATIENT: What kind of accident?
FRIEND: An automobile accident.
PATIENT: Was it bad?
FRIEND: Very bad, I'm afraid.
PATIENT: What happened to my car?
FRIEND: Ah, asking the important questions first, I see.
PATIENT: Those wheels meant a lot to me.
FRIEND: Apparently so.
PATIENT: Well, what happened to it?

FRIEND: Your automobile?
PATIENT: Yes.
FRIEND: As they say in the vernacular, it was "totaled."
PATIENT: Oh, no! How'd it happen?
FRIEND: You don't remember?
PATIENT: Not a thing.
FRIEND: Driving too fast on a rain-slick street, you missed a curve, bounced off a tree, then wrapped yourself around a utility pole.
PATIENT: Wow!
FRIEND: Wow, indeed. The neighborhood was really upset. Your accident blacked out some important television sporting event or other at a very critical moment of play.
PATIENT: You mean that's all they cared about—some game!
FRIEND: There's no accounting for people's tastes or values sometimes.
PATIENT: You can say that again.
FRIEND: I don't like to repeat myself. Anyway, they had to use the Jaws-of-Life to extricate you from the wreck. (*The* FRIEND *laughs to himself.*)
PATIENT: What's so funny?
FRIEND: Sorry, I was just thinking what an oxymoron that phrase is.
PATIENT: What phrase?
FRIEND: "Jaws-of-Life." It's like "jumbo shrimp" or "single family home." In any case, they pried you loose from the car and brought you here.
PATIENT: Was—was anyone else hurt?
FRIEND: Ah, now you're getting to the really important questions.
PATIENT: Well, was there? I'm worried about my car insurance and all.
FRIEND: (*disappointed*) Oh, that. I see. Well, if that's all you're worried about, no one else was hurt.
PATIENT: Whew! That's a relief.
FRIEND: Yes. I'm sure it is.
PATIENT: Not that I'd want anyone else hurt, you understand.
FRIEND: Of course not. (*The* PATIENT *begins checking himself over.*)
PATIENT: Hey, I thought you said I was in a pretty bad accident.
FRIEND: You were.
PATIENT: Then why don't I have any broken bones or bruises and that kind of stuff?
FRIEND: Oh, you did: multiple lacerations, broken arm, broken leg, several rib fractures, not to mention a number of internal injuries delicacy prevents me from going into at the moment. In short, you were a mess. Over time, however, the healing process works wonders.

PATIENT: Over time? You mean . . .

FRIEND: Yes. You've been here for quite some time.

PATIENT: How long?

FRIEND: Quite awhile.

PATIENT: Could you be more precise?

FRIEND: Let me put it this way. Remember that car stereo system you were so proud of?

PATIENT: Sure. Eight-track stereo quadraphonic. Yeah, what about it?

FRIEND: Now it's a collector's item.

PATIENT: That long?

FRIEND: Yes.

PATIENT: Was I in some kind of coma or something?

FRIEND: Were and still are. It's irreversible.

PATIENT: You mean I'm brain dead?

FRIEND: Not exactly.

PATIENT: (*laughing*) My teachers used to say I was brain dead. (*dawning on him*) Hey, wait a minute.

FRIEND: Yes?

PATIENT: Well, if I'm supposed to be in a coma, how am I able to talk to you?

FRIEND: I'm special.

PATIENT: And that's why you're wearing that weird outfit.

FRIEND: It's not so weird. Besides, it's company issue.

PATIENT: Are you some kind of guardian angel?

FRIEND: Not exactly.

PATIENT: I always pictured guardian angels with robes and wings.

FRIEND: Some people picture them wearing berets and patrolling city streets.

PATIENT: Huh?

FRIEND: Never mind.

PATIENT: Well, if you're not an angel, then what are you?

FRIEND: Company policy does not allow me to discuss theology — or politics, for that matter — with my clients.

PATIENT: I'm your client?

FRIEND: Yes, in a manner of speaking. In fact, you're my only client.

PATIENT: Really? Why's that?

FRIEND: Company policy. We're only allowed one client at a time. Usually, the relationship is short-term, but there are exceptional cases.

PATIENT: Like mine.

FRIEND: Yes. At the moment of expiration —
PATIENT: You mean death.
FRIEND: Like many of you, we eschew such vulgarities. Anyway, at the moment of expiration, it is our task to lead the disembodied neophyte to the other side. In your case, they used extraordinary means to preserve your life, so here I am still waiting for you to, uh —
PATIENT: Expire?
FRIEND: Precisely. Then I'll finally be able to escort you to the other side.
PATIENT: The other side — I've always wondered what that's like.
FRIEND: Believe me, you're not the only one.
PATIENT: What's it like on the other side?
FRIEND: I'm afraid I cannot discuss that with anyone who is not fully disembodied.
PATIENT: Don't tell me: company policy.
FRIEND: As a matter of fact, yes.
PATIENT: Oh, come on. You can at least give me a little hint, can't you? (*The* FRIEND *turns his back.*) At least tell me if it's better than we have here.
FRIEND: (*turning around*) Far better, I assure you.
PATIENT: Then what are we waiting for? Let's go.

(*The* PATIENT *tries to get out of bed, but finds himself held back by the feeding tube.*)

PATIENT: What's this?
FRIEND: A feeding tube. A gastric feeding tube, to be precise. It is what has been keeping you alive, such as it is.
PATIENT: Well, I'll just take it off, and we'll be on our way. Okay? (*The* FRIEND *shakes his head.*) Hey, I can't get it off.
FRIEND: No, and you won't be able to.
PATIENT: But I don't understand. It's my body. I've got my rights.
FRIEND: Sorry to say, you lost those rights when you went into a coma. You've put your fate in the hands of others.
PATIENT: You mean my mom and dad.
FRIEND: Yes. You were very wise in deciding to give power of attorney to your parents at such a young age.
PATIENT: It was my dad's idea. I didn't want to bother with a will. You know how it is when you're young.
FRIEND: Personally? No, I can't say that I do, but I imagine that you feel rather invincible, don't you?

PATIENT: Yeah, that's it. Invincible.

FRIEND: That you personally are never going to expire.

PATIENT: That's what I thought all right. But the old man was right for a change. I've got to hand it to him this time. Only—

FRIEND: Only what?

PATIENT: Only, if I've given mom and dad the power of attorney, what's taking them so long to—to—

FRIEND: Let you go?

PATIENT: Yeah.

FRIEND: Well, there's the rub, as one of your poets was fond of saying. Though you gave your parents power of attorney to manage your financial affairs, you never specified how far they should go with your medical treatment.

PATIENT: Well, I'm sure I've mentioned my views on that issue once in awhile.

FRIEND: To your parents?

PATIENT: I think so.

FRIEND: Or was it to your friends at a college fraternity party one night when you had, shall we say, imbibed a bit too much?

PATIENT: Hey, how do you know so much about me?

FRIEND: Waiting around so long, I've had the luxury of reviewing your records.

PATIENT: And I thought the IRS was bad. You mean to tell me my parents aren't going to pull the plug on me?

FRIEND: Indelicately put, but yes, that's it in a nutshell.

PATIENT: You think they would know better. You think they would know what I want, what's best for me.

FRIEND: Oh, I think your father does. He just doesn't want to upset your mother.

PATIENT: What's Mom's problem?

FRIEND: She still thinks you're going to come out of your coma.

PATIENT: After all this time?

FRIEND: Apparently, yes.

PATIENT: So I'm stuck here, is that it?

FRIEND: That makes two of us.

PATIENT: Now what do I do?

FRIEND: Don't you mean "we"?

PATIENT: All right. What do *we* do?

FRIEND: We wait.

PATIENT: That's it? We just wait?

FRIEND: Yes, until either your mother comes to grips with her emotions or it comes time for you to—

PATIENT: Expire?

FRIEND: Yes.

PATIENT: And what does your crystal ball tell you about how long either event will take?

FRIEND: Oh, the company doesn't issue us crystal balls.

PATIENT: You know what I mean.

FRIEND: I do not have access to either scenario. It's—

PATIENT AND FRIEND: (*together*) Company policy.

PATIENT: Well, I've never been one for waiting around!

FRIEND: Witness your automobile.

PATIENT: There must be something that can be done!

FRIEND: Now look what I've done. I've gotten you upset. I should never have woken you up. What will my supervisor say?

PATIENT: There's got to be a way! There— (*beginning to tire out*) there has to be.

FRIEND: All of this has been too much for you, my boy. Why don't you just lie back and rest for awhile.

PATIENT: Yeah, I guess I am a little tired all of a sudden.

(*The* PATIENT *props the pillows up behind his back and lies back.*)

FRIEND: That's it. Just rest yourself.

(*The* FRIEND *moves to stage right, looks at his tabloid again briefly, then suddenly looks up.*)

FRIEND: There is someone coming.

PATIENT: (*turning his head left*) Who is it?

FRIEND: I believe it is your mother.

PATIENT: My mother!

FRIEND: Yes. She's right on time.

(*The* MOTHER *enters from left. She carries a bouquet of fresh flowers. She stops for a moment midway between the entrance and the bed and looks at her son.*)

PATIENT: Mom!

FRIEND: She can't hear you.

PATIENT: Mom, it's me!

FRIEND: I told you she can't hear you.

PATIENT: (*to the* FRIEND) Why not?

FRIEND: No one on this side can hear you. As far as she knows, you're still curled up in a fetal position.

PATIENT: That's not fair!

FRIEND: I'll be sure to take that up with the proper authorities.

(*The* MOTHER *sighs, goes over to the night table, and puts the bouquet into a vase.*)

PATIENT: She's changed so much.

FRIEND: Yes, that happens over time.

(MOTHER *goes to the left side of the bed and looks down at her son, not "seeing" him in the same way that we have.*)

MOTHER: And how are you today, son? (*The* PATIENT *is about to answer her, but the* FRIEND *cautions him.*)

FRIEND: Shh!

MOTHER: Your father will be along in a few minutes. I asked him to stop by the gift shop and pick up a new novel for you. (*She begins stroking his hair.*)

PATIENT: (*to the* FRIEND) New novel? What's she talking about?

FRIEND: Every day your mother sits by your bedside and reads you several chapters from a book.

PATIENT: I hate reading. I always have.

FRIEND: Well, despite your aversion, you've become quite the literary connoisseur. Dickens, Hawthorne, and Hemingway have all become your boon companions — that is, without your knowing about it, of course.

PATIENT: Same old Mom. She majored in English at college.

FRIEND: It's strange, though.

PATIENT: What's so strange about her being an English major?

FRIEND: No, what I mean is your mother has a strange penchant for editing the texts to her own liking.

PATIENT: What do you mean?

FRIEND: In the versions she reads to you, Little Nell in *The Old Curiosity Shop,* Catherine in *A Farewell to Arms* — the lot of them never seem to — well, expire.

(*The* MOTHER *pulls up a chair and sits by the side of the bed.*)

MOTHER: Did I tell you the latest? Your cousin Becky just got engaged.
PATIENT: (*to the* FRIEND) Becky's hardly ten.
FRIEND: They do grow up fast, don't they? She's eighteen now.
MOTHER: Let's see, what else? Oh, you won't believe this. Your Aunt Audrey is getting married again.
PATIENT: That's her third.
FRIEND: Correction: her fifth.
PATIENT: What!
MOTHER: And I already told you your cousin Annie's pregnant again.

(*The* FRIEND *opens, closes, and opens his hand.*)

PATIENT: Her tenth! (*The* FRIEND *nods.*) I don't believe this!
MOTHER: (*standing*) Well, I guess it's time for your exercises.
PATIENT: What's she talking about?
FRIEND: You'll see.

(*The* MOTHER *grabs her son's leg, pushes it toward him, then away from him repeatedly. He offers no resistance.*)

MOTHER: Remember when you were a swimmer at Central, how you were always doing calisthenics. You seemed to eat and breathe nothing else.
PATIENT: I was quite the jock.
FRIEND: So I've heard.
MOTHER: Then every day before and after school and on weekends you'd swim laps. Back and forth, you'd go, back and forth, endlessly it seemed. I don't know how you did it.
PATIENT: Neither did I.
MOTHER: And now this. Also endless. I don't know how you do it. I don't know how I do it.

(*She puts his leg down, then she sits down. She puts her head on the bed and cries softly.*)

PATIENT: She's crying.
FRIEND: Yes. It's been a painful and prolonged ordeal for her.
PATIENT: I've only seen her cry once before, when my grandfather died. This can't go on. She's got to be made to understand it's no use. She can't go on this way. (*to the* MOTHER) Mom—Mom. Don't cry. Please.

FRIEND: She can't hear you.
PATIENT: (*angrily*) She's got to hear me! You just butt out for once!
FRIEND: All right, suit yourself.
PATIENT: (*to the* MOTHER) Mom, are you listening? (*The* FRIEND *shakes his head.*) You got to stop doing this to yourself. And you've got to let me go. I want to go. Understand? Look, remember that time you didn't want me to go on that hiking trip by myself down the Appalachian Trail. You were so worried and all. But you gave in, and you let me go. Everything turned out all right, didn't it? Well, there's another trip, a much more important trip I have to go on, and you have to — you hear me? — you have to let me go. Mom, can you hear me? Mom? (*He turns away.*) Oh, what's the use?

(*A man in his 50s, the* FATHER, *enters from the left, carrying a small paper bag. He stops when he sees his wife crying, then goes over to her, and places his hand gently on her shoulder.*)

FATHER: Are you all right, dear?
PATIENT: (*turning around*) Dad?
MOTHER: Oh, I'm fine. I just got a little tired after getting Sonny started on his exercise, that's all.
PATIENT: (*to the* FRIEND) I always hated that nickname.
FRIEND: Yes. I can see why. Awfully generic, isn't it?
MOTHER: (*about to get up*) Well, I better do his other leg.
FATHER: No, dear. You rest. I'll do it.
PATIENT: (*to the* FRIEND) My God, when did the old man become so caring and considerate?
FRIEND: It comes naturally to some people. Others learn it the hard way — through tragedy and misfortune.
FATHER: Oh, I almost forgot; here's the novel you wanted.
MOTHER: Thank you, dear.

(*The* FATHER *goes over to the other side of the bed and begins exercising his son's leg. The* MOTHER *takes a paperback out of the bag and stares at it.*)

MOTHER: What's this?
FATHER: What's what?
MOTHER: This book.
FATHER: Something wrong with it?
MOTHER: It's trash.

(Even though he can't be seen, the FRIEND *quickly hides the tabloid behind his back.)*

FATHER: So?
MOTHER: I asked you to pick up a classic.
FATHER: The lady at the gift shop said it's been on the bestseller list for months.
MOTHER: That doesn't make it a classic.
FATHER: It's a gift shop, not a library. What did you expect? Anyway, I liked the cover, full of sex and violence.
PATIENT: Way to go, Dad!
MOTHER: I can't read this rubbish to our son.
FATHER: Why not?
PATIENT: Yeah, why not?
FATHER: If anything's going to snap him out of his coma maybe that piece of trash will, instead of all those boring old books you keep reading him.
PATIENT: That's not fair! *(to the* FRIEND*)* I thought you said he'd changed?
FRIEND: Sometimes he slips back into his old ways. He's only human, as your species likes to say.

(Silence. The MOTHER *puts the book on the night table. The* FATHER *stops exercising his son's leg.)*

FATHER: I'm sorry, dear. I didn't mean that.
MOTHER: That's all right.
FATHER: You're not mad at me, are you?
MOTHER: I don't think so.
FATHER: You don't sound convinced. Look, I said what I did because I just don't know how long this can go on.
MOTHER: As long as it takes.
FATHER: That may be forever.
MOTHER: Then so be it.
FATHER: Look at us. All we do is arrange our lives around hospital visits. We never go out anymore. Never see anyone. When's the last time we took a vacation?
MOTHER: I don't care. All I want is to be here when my baby wakes up.
PATIENT: Baby!
FATHER: Baby!

FRIEND: There must be an echo in here.

FATHER: He's thirty-five years old, for God's sake.

MOTHER: He's still my little baby to me.

FATHER: Let's face it. He's not getting any better, and we're only getting worse. It's hopeless.

MOTHER: Don't say that.

FATHER: Well, somebody's got to say it.

MOTHER: No, no. One of these days he's going to open his eyes, sit up, and talk to us.

FATHER: After all this time?

MOTHER: Of course. It's happened to lots of people just like him. Just the other day, there was that case in the papers.

FATHER: But maybe our son's case is different. Then he'll just linger here, just like he has for years. Maybe it's time to let him go. Maybe that's what he'd want us to do.

PATIENT: Tell her, Dad!

MOTHER: No, I can't let him go. I won't. You don't understand. He was so full of promise. His business was just starting to take off. And then that terrible accident had to happen.

PATIENT: (*to the* FRIEND) I was quite the entrepreneur.

FRIEND: Humility hangs heavy on your shoulders.

FATHER: You forget. I had high hopes for him too. And I—I always wanted grandchildren, of course.

PATIENT: Marriage—kids. I'm not so sure I was ready for it then, but down the line—sure.

FATHER: There's something else we better discuss, too.

MOTHER: What's that?

FATHER: Our medical benefits have run out, we've been dipping into our savings, and before you know it, there'll be nothing left for us in our old age.

PATIENT: (*to the* FRIEND) Is that true?

FRIEND: Unfortunately, yes.

MOTHER: I don't care about the money. It would have been his eventually anyway.

FATHER: Well, you better start caring about it soon, or we're going to find ourselves living on the streets.

PATIENT: (*to the* FRIEND) That doesn't happen anymore, does it?

FRIEND: Today? More than you could ever imagine.

(The FATHER *goes over to his wife's side.)*

FATHER: I'm sorry, dear. I never meant to upset you, but I just think it's time we began looking at this thing from a practical standpoint.

MOTHER: Believe me, I'm trying to. I really am. It's easier for you; you've always been the pragmatic one.

PATIENT: (*to the* FRIEND) You see who I take after.

FRIEND: The apple never falls far from the tree.

FATHER: I just think we should be preparing ourselves for the inevitable, that's all.

MOTHER: Well, we have a difference of opinion on what's inevitable, don't we?

(Just then the DOCTOR, *30-ish, enters from the left, carrying the* PATIENT'S *chart.)*

DOCTOR: Hello, there.

MOTHER: Hello, Doctor.

FATHER: Hello.

DOCTOR: I'm sorry to intrude.

MOTHER: That's quite all right, Doctor.

DOCTOR: I was just making my rounds; thought I'd drop by to see how your son is doing.

FATHER: By all means, do.

DOCTOR: Thank you.

(The DOCTOR *examines the* PATIENT *and refers to the chart while the* PARENTS *look on.)*

PATIENT: (*to the* FRIEND) This guy looks awfully young to be a doctor.

FRIEND: That makes you even. You look awfully young to be a patient.

PATIENT: You think he knows what he's doing?

FRIEND: To a certain extent they all do.

MOTHER: So how's he doing, Doctor?

FRIEND: About the same.

MOTHER: No better, no worse?

DOCTOR: No, about the same.

FATHER: (*angry*) "About the same" — that's what you said last week, and the week before that. As far back as I can remember that's all you doctors have been saying.

DOCTOR: I'm sorry, I don't know what else I can say.

MOTHER: Don't mind my husband, Doctor, he's been having one of his days.

PATIENT: He used to have them a lot.

DOCTOR: That's all right. I understand. Both of you have been through a very long ordeal.

FATHER: I'm sorry, Doctor. I didn't mean to fly off the handle like that.

DOCTOR: It's all right, believe me.

FATHER: It's just that my wife and I were just discussing—actually we were arguing—the pros and cons about, you know, continuing treatment for our son.

MOTHER: I think we should still continue it, Doctor.

FATHER: And I'm for discontinuing it. What do you think, Doctor?

DOCTOR: Well, I don't know what to tell you. It's a difficult decision.

PATIENT: (*to the* FRIEND) He's a big help.

FATHER: May I ask you a question?

DOCTOR: Yes, of course.

FATHER: If our son's coma were irreversible, wouldn't it be better for everyone concerned just to let him go?

DOCTOR: Yes, I suppose it would. And fortunately, in this state, your decision would not be challenged since you have power of attorney.

PATIENT: Listen to the man!

MOTHER: But you don't know whether his coma is irreversible or not, do you, Doctor?

PATIENT: Mom, what are you doing?

DOCTOR: No, we don't.

FATHER: Not even after all this time?

DOCTOR: No, our medical skill only goes so far. I'm sorry. I can see this is going to take more soul-searching and discussion before you two can come to a consensus. (*looking at his watch*) Well, if you'll excuse me, it's time I finished making my rounds.

MOTHER: Of course, Doctor.

DOCTOR: Goodbye.

FATHER: Goodbye.

MOTHER: Goodbye, Doctor. (*The* DOCTOR *exits.*)

PATIENT: (*to the* FRIEND) Well, it looks like we're back to square one.

FRIEND: Yes, unfortunately.

FATHER: Dear, there's something else I've been meaning to bring up for some time.

MOTHER: What is it? You might as well get it off your chest, too.

FATHER: Well, I think we should be thinking about what we want done when our time comes.

MOTHER: When our time comes to do what?

FATHER: You know, to shuffle off our mortal coils and all that.

FRIEND: Very tastefully put!

MOTHER: I'd rather not discuss that topic right now, if you don't mind.

FATHER: Well, we're going to have to someday. The only sure thing in life people put off talking about is their own demise. (*He takes several brochures from his jacket.*)

MOTHER: What are those?

FATHER: Brochures.

MOTHER: What kind of brochures?

FATHER: Brochures I sent away for. They came in the mail this morning. They're from this Right-to-Die group.

MOTHER: Last week it was from some radical environmental group that said we should stop mowing our lawn. What next?

FATHER: They're nothing like that. Listen, they suggest we make out a living will or name a proxy to let people know exactly what our wishes are if, God forbid, we should wind up like — well, you know.

MOTHER: This is all a little morbid, isn't it?

FATHER: Not at all. Look, if I've learned anything in the past few years, it's that if it were me in that bed like that, I wouldn't want my life prolonged by extraordinary means. No, sir. And I'd be sure to honor your wishes, whatever they were. Only, we have to put them in writing, you understand. The sooner, the better.

FRIEND: Eminent advice, I must say.

FATHER: Please, will you take a look at the brochures?

MOTHER: I can't look at them now. I'll — I'll look at them some other time.

FATHER: You promise.

MOTHER: Yes, I promise.

FATHER: Good!

MOTHER: Now put them away.

FATHER: Okay, if you insist. (*He puts the brochures away.*) Are you going to read to him for awhile?

MOTHER: Not that trash you bought.

FATHER: Oh. Tell you what, I'll drive you down to the library where you can pick out something you like. What do you say?

MOTHER: I'd say it's a very good idea.

FATHER: Good. Then let's go.

MOTHER: Wait a minute. (*kissing her son's forehead*) Goodbye, son. We'll be back in a little bit.

PATIENT: (*looking into her eyes*) Mom, you gotta stop doing this to yourself, understand? More important, you've gotta stop doing this to me. (*She goes over to her husband.*) Dad, try and talk some sense into her, will ya?

(*Arm in arm, the* MOTHER *and the* FATHER *leave the room slowly.*)

PATIENT: (*yawning*) Well, I guess, as they say, that's that.
FRIEND: Yes, for the time being. You sound tired.
PATIENT: I'm exhausted.
FRIEND: Then why don't you try and get a little sleep?
PATIENT: (*yawning again*) That seems to be all I've been doing for a very long time.
FRIEND: That's all right. Some people need more sleep than others.
PATIENT: I guess I could use a little shut-eye at that. You'll be here when I wake up, won't you?
FRIEND: Don't worry. I'm not going anywhere.
PATIENT: Goodnight then.
FRIEND: Goodnight.

(*The* PATIENT *falls asleep, gradually reverting to the fetal position we saw him in at the beginning of the play.*)

FRIEND: "Good night, sweet prince, / And flights of angels sing thee to thy rest!" (ANOTHER FRIEND *enters from the left.*)
ANOTHER FRIEND: Hello again, Friend.
FRIEND: Hello again. How did the highway accident go?
ANOTHER FRIEND: Not too well. My client's been moved to intensive care.
FRIEND: Sorry to hear it. Good luck.
ANOTHER FRIEND: Thanks. (ANOTHER FRIEND *exits.*)
FRIEND: Believe me, you're going to need it. The case sounds awfully familiar.

(*He notices the trashy novel on the night table. Curious, he picks the book up and skims through it.*)

FRIEND: Hmm, it seems like an awfully long read. (*He sits down next to the bed.*) But it appears as though I have plenty of time — plenty of time. (*He settles in for a good read.*)

THE LIGHTS FADE
END OF PLAY

Commentary

The fact that all the characters in CE McClelland's *Time to Go* are generic — the Mother, the Father, the Friend, the Patient, the Doctor — tells us something about the universality (given modern medical technology) of the comatose patient hooked up to mechanical devices that could keep him or her alive indefinitely. The play begins when the Patient, in a coma for eight years following an automobile accident, is awakened by "the Friend," the drily witty guide who waits — somewhat impatiently — to conduct him to the "other side." Together, Patient and Friend observe the Father and the Mother, who struggle with the various issues — emotional, moral, financial — that accompany termination of treatment.

The theme of the patient who suddenly wakes up out of a coma precisely parallels an important case in the history of legislation about informed consent in regard to incompetent patients. Karen Ann Quinlan was a young New Jersey woman who in 1975 was put on life support systems. Her parents, convinced that their daughter would never recover consciousness, asked that life support be discontinued. Though their request was turned down by the hospital, the New Jersey Supreme Court eventually decided in favor of the parents. In arriving at this decision — the first legal case about life support ever adjudicated — the court imagined what Karen would want, were she to become "miraculously lucid for an interval" and able to "effectively decide upon discontinuance of the life-support apparatus, even if it meant the prospect of natural death."* This is precisely what happens in *Time to Go*. The patient who suddenly comes out of a coma, able to understand his or her situation fully, is an exact parallel to the doctrine of "substituted judgment," used in the *Quinlan* case to explain how proxies should decide for patients.

The play is built on two fantasies: the one ancient, the personification of Death as a messenger or guide; the other more modern, the belief that people in a coma are able to hear the voices of those speaking in the room and that they have wishes and desires but are unable to communicate them. McClelland sets the whimsical tone of *Time to Go* with the play's opening lines: "'Elvis and Marilyn spotted in honeymoon hot tub.' . . . 'Vice President is alien imposter.'" The relevance of the tabloid headlines is obvious: the comatose Patient resembles Marilyn Monroe and Elvis Presley, whom we never are quite willing to let die, while the Friend himself, like the

---

In the matter of Karen Quinlan 70 N.J. 10, 355 A.2d 647 (1976), at 663.

unnamed Vice President (the play was written at the end of the Quayle era)
is an "alien," if not an "imposter." The Patient's initial response on waking
up to the world of the play is to express surprise at the presence of this
strange figure; later on he asks whether the Friend is a guardian angel. "Not
exactly," is the reply. Dressed in a white tuxedo rather than robe and wings,
the Friend is not the traditional guardian angel who might presumably have
tried to avert the Patient's accident. Nor is he one of the real-life "guardian
angels" who patrol city streets wearing berets.

The allusions to supernatural and urban protectors exemplify the way
the play blends the surreal and the matter-of-fact while consistently deflat-
ing and demythologizing its supernatural premise. The Friend is a visitor
from another plane of being whose white tuxedo is "company issue," who
reads tabloid newspapers, and who can never bring himself to use the word
"death." What, then, are we to make of this figure? The answer is that the
Friend is a convention. The role goes back to the figure of Death in the
medieval morality play, who summons the soul of Everyman to the afterworld; and beyond this to the mythological figure of Hermes Psychopompos, who conducts the souls of the dead to Hades. Hermes is a playful
god, a thief and trickster, whose youth and high spirits contrast with his
more somber role as psychopomp, and we find the same paradoxical blend
of tones in McClelland's play. But the differences between McClelland's
"Friend" and the figures of Death and Hermes Psychopompos are so great
as to make their kinship a comic one. There is no awe, threat, or sense of the
numinous about the Friend in *Time to Go*. In this modern habit of stripping
death of its mystery, McClelland's play resembles *Here Comes Mr. Jordan*,
where Death appears as a vaguely benevolent and sometimes faintly comic
figure; or the 1946 British film, *A Matter of Life and Death*, where the
"Heavenly Messenger" appears in a beret and a curious, anachronistic
costume to summon the protagonist to the afterworld; or *Heaven Can
Wait*, where Death is personified as a man in a business suit whom Gramps
can trap in an apple tree until his conditions — that his young grandson
survive — are satisfied. Death in *Time to Go* can likewise be kept at bay by
modern medical technology: the sense of inevitable doom and fate in its
medieval or renaissance incarnations is replaced here by the frustrations and
uncertainties of choice.

In such modern fictions the supernatural suggestions of a divine order
and an afterlife are stripped from the figure of Death or psychopomp. While
there is an "other side" that is "far better" than our own in *Time to Go,* the
play, like the Friend, refuses to bring up theology: "company policy" does

not allow it. The Father and Mother are not helped to a decision by any religious sense that death is not final or that their son would be better off in heaven. No judgment is passed on the life of the young man himself, or on his soul (the play gives us no indication that he even has a soul). The Friend's resistance to discussions of theology (or politics) with his client typifies the play's consistent refusal to allow its premise to become anything more than a premise. All we know about the "other side" is that it is governed by "company policy" and administered by "supervisors." At the same time that it deprives death of religious associations, the play is severely devoid of nostalgia or of wishful thinking. The young man, revived to the world of the play, is able to reconsider his present and his past, but this serves no real purpose: he does not change, and even if he did, we sense that this would make no difference to his future. Trapped by medical technology between the worlds of the living and the dead, he cannot do or say anything. In a sense, advance medical directives are a response to the new Limbo modern technology has created between the states of life and death. They may not permit us to return to the world of the living, but they do enable us to pass over to "the other side."

The play combines comic whimsy with a dry and severe realism. This balance is evident even in its symmetrical structure. The play begins and ends with brief scenes that both establish the supernatural frame of the action and — by the odd but distinctly worldly dress of the two Friends and their cheery greetings and businesslike behavior — strip it of supernatural aura. These opening and closing episodes of dialogue between the two Friends bracket the "supernatural" scene between the Patient and the Friend with its predominantly comic tone, despite some darker touches, and the "realistic" scene between the Father and the Mother, whose tone, while still touched with comedy, is serious and at moments even grim. The transition between the two scenes is smoothed by allowing Patient and Friend to comment on the dialogue between Father and Mother; at the same time the stern separation of two worlds is emphasized by the fact that the Mother cannot see that her son is alive and conscious and that the Patient cannot make his mother hear his frantic pleas. Whatever the Patient may have learned in his brief traffic with the other side cannot be communicated to those who need it most; the supernatural premise does nothing to alter or ease the parents' real dilemma.

This strict division between Beyond and Here is paralleled by the division between the characters: not only between the Friend and the Patient on one side and the parents on the other but also for each of these pairs. The Friend, bowing to "company policy," never communicates even his own limited knowledge to the Patient. When the Patient asks the Friend if anyone else was hurt in the automobile accident and the Friend remarks approvingly, "Now you're getting to the really important questions," it would seem that the stage is set for some sort of moral learning. But there is no moral learning in this play, and when the patient responds with a comment about his insurance coverage, we laugh. Similarly, the Mother and the Father seem unable to communicate with each other. The Mother is locked into her sentimental conviction that her son — "my baby" — will eventually come out of the coma; and the Father seems unable to convince her that it is unlikely their son will ever recover, that their financial resources are nearly exhausted, and that their marriage is under considerable strain.

With this absence of real communication or interaction goes a sense of the isolation of each character. The Patient is more concerned with the fate of his automobile than with anyone else who might have been injured in the accident. The Doctor and the Friend are uncomfortably similar in certain ways. Both are trapped by the circumstances of the Patient's death-in-life, both answer questions evasively, both are concerned to get on with the next patient or the next job. Like the Friend, the Doctor has access to higher knowledge — scientific rather than supernatural — but he seems equally un- willing or unable to communicate it. For the Mother, the son she thinks she loves is really not an independent individual but "my baby," his present fetal position and gastric feeding tube emphasizing her reluctance to allow him to separate from her by either birth or death. Her love of literature does not, like the poems in *Journey Into That Good Night,* help her to come to terms with mortality, either her own or others'; rather she edits the texts, both in life and literature, to cut out the ending she does not want to face. The exercises she performs, pushing her son's leg back and forth "endlessly," typify not only the failure of real contact and interaction between them but also the empty monotony of a life that consists of mere repetition — more children for Cousin Anne, more husbands for Aunt Audrey — lived without any sense of an ending.

In this bleak vista the Father seems the most hopeful figure. He is the only character who seems truly to touch another: he "places his hand gently on [the Mother's] shoulder." Unlike his son, he has learned something through tragedy and misfortune: he has even become "caring and consider- ate," as his son observes. In contrast to the Friend, who eschews such "vulgarities" as the word "die," the Father is willing and able to speak bluntly about his son's death: "somebody's got to say it," he observes.

Moreover, he is free from the literary pretensions shared by his wife and by the Friend, who admires Shakespeare while actually enjoying tabloids and the sensational novel that the Father picks out. The Father's taste for "sex and violence" is grounded in vitality and a love of life, and this encourages us to believe that he has the force and the passion finally to persuade his wife to discuss the topics she would like to repress or deny.

But the play at its conclusion does not permit us a sense of resolution, and this is evident in the last lines or actions of each of the characters. The Doctor offers no help at all. Rather than sitting down with these parents and helping them talk about their dilemma, he or she leaves the Patient's room to finish rounds, abandoning them to "more soul-searching and discussion." Though Father and Mother exit (according to the stage directions) "arm in arm," the fact that they are headed toward a library to try and find a classic to the Mother's taste is a measure of the slim likelihood that they will come to any resolution about their son. The play twice alludes to Hamlet's famous soliloquy, in which the Prince longs to "shuffle off this mortal coil," but exclaims "Ay, there's the rub!" as he recalls the dreams that may come after the sleep of death. The Friend's final remark to the Patient, as he goes back to his endless sleep, is likewise a quotation from *Hamlet:* "Good night, sweet prince / And flights of angels sing thee to thy rest." For those who recognize the quotation — it is Horatio's leave-taking of the dead Hamlet near the end of that play — it is a deeply ironic allusion. The irony derives not only from the marked contrast between Hamlet and the Patient and between Horatio and the Friend — the heroic and non-heroic — but also because of a thematic similarity. Shakespeare's play is about a young man who could not decide whether "to be or not to be"; the problem in McClelland's contemporary play of indecision is not the going, it seems, but the letting go. Meanwhile, as the Friend tells the Patient — "We wait" — and the echo of Beckett's *Waiting for Godot* is surely not accidental. As a nice parallel to the parents' quest for a classic, in the final action of the play the Friend with evident delight picks up the "bestseller" left by the Father, remarking, "It seems like an awfully long read. . . . But, it appears as though I have plenty of time — plenty of time."

Suggestions for Performance and Discussion

The play opens with four characters seated, from left to right: the Friend, the Patient, the Mother, the Father. The Patient's head is bowed to indicate that he is asleep; the Friend is reading his newspaper; the Mother and the

Father face away from the audience. The Other Friend and the Doctor are seated close to but not with the rest of the cast.

PROPS
A packet of advance directives (or some substitute), a copy of a tabloid newspaper such as the *National Enquirer,* a novel with a racy picture or title.

CASTING
The success of this play will turn on how well one is able to cast the Friend and the Patient. While the Mother and the Father are important roles, the performance will succeed even if these are played by weaker actors.

The Friend. This character is sophisticated, polished, condescending but affable, and could be slightly mannered. The Friend has a dry but lively sense of humor, and the actor must be able to project this. This part could be played by a man or a woman.

The Patient. He is brash, natural and spontaneous, impulsive — as he himself says, a "jock." His rough-hewn personality contrasts with the smoothness of the Friend. In auditions, this actor should certainly read some of the Patient's dialogue with the Friend, but also the important speech where he pleads with his mother to let him go (just before the Father's entrance).

The Mother. She is sentimental but stubborn. The success of this part depends on the actress's ability to display grief: just after she does her son's exercises and just before the Father's entrance she "puts her head on the bed and cries softly." Auditions for the part should include this passage. Her emotion is important to the shift of tone from the humorous exchange between the Friend and the Patient to the seriousness of the parents' dialogue. To the extent that she can engage us with her grieving, she will be a more sympathetic character, and the conflict between the parents will become more complex and more interesting.

The Father. The play suggests that the Father has been changed in important ways by the tragedy of his son's condition: when he offers to exercise his son's other leg, the Patient exclaims, "My God, when did the old man become so caring and considerate?" The actor playing the Father must be able to suggest earlier traits of crudity, practicality, and forthrightness, which he shares with his son — their shared taste for "sex and violence," for example — as well a new consideration and tact directed here toward the Mother.

The Doctor. This role evokes different interpretations, and is best cast with a medical student, who will benefit most from the experience of "playing" a physician. The actor or director must decide whether to make this character chilly, distant, and professional, or warm but helpless. Perhaps the best solution may be to try for an ambiguity which will allow the audience to decide whether the Doctor is at fault or whether he or she does all that is possible to help. This role can be played by a male or female actor.

Another Friend. This very minor role (which can also be played by a male or a female actor) is useful for including in performances certain kinds of health care professionals (physicians, social workers, or chaplains) who may not have the time to undertake larger roles and who may not have acting experience or talent.

STAGING

The Mother and the Father turn away from the audience when not on stage. The Doctor and Another Friend actually enter and leave the acting area, remaining standing while they speak: this helps make the staging more dynamic and varied. But these actors must be careful to face toward the audience enough to be heard.

Just before her exit, when the Mother says goodbye to her son, instead of "kissing her son's forehead" (McClelland's stage directions), which would be awkward in a reading performance, our director had her take her son's hand, kiss it, and hold it up to her cheek.

Early in the play, when McClelland's stage directions indicate that "the Patient tries to get out of bed, but finds himself held back by the feeding tube," the actor stands up and mimes discovery of a feeding tube, trying to pull it away from him. In reading performances, gestures like this (or the Mother's exercise routine) are very effective precisely because they are so few.

The Friend hints at a hypnotic or magical gesture when he puts the Patient to sleep, just before the Mother's entrance. At the end of the play, the Friend displays considerable interest in the popular novel with its "sex and violence," reaching across the Patient to pick it up at the end of the play. As he begins to read it, he settles himself comfortably for the long wait ahead.

DISCUSSION QUESTIONS — GENERAL

1. Why does it seem so hard for us to let go of our loved ones (or our patients) at the end of life? Do we find this difficult because of our concern for the dying person, or are there other reasons?

   2. *It proved valuable during discussion to ask the medical student playing the*

Doctor about his or her experience acting this role. We then asked the audience: How did you respond to the Doctor? If you were in the place of the Mother or the Father, would you want this physician as your son's doctor? Why, or why not? Should he/she take a more active role in helping the parents with their decision? Should the physician offer his/her own opinion as to what the parents should do in a case such as this? What might the Doctor have said or done to be more helpful?

3. *To the Mother:* What helped you portray this character? What sort of person do you imagine the Mother to be? *To the audience:* What do you think would enable the Mother to accept the fact that her son is not going to come out of his coma and to let him go? What kind of background and what experiences can explain her adopting this kind of attitude toward a son who has been in a coma for so long?

4. Have the parents changed in relation to each other as a result of their son's long illness? What other resources might the parents turn to for help in dealing with this experience?

5. In the play, the Father brings up, as a reason for allowing their son to die, the fact that they have nearly exhausted their financial resources. Do you think monetary considerations should influence decisions about whether or not comatose patients should remain on life support systems?

6. How many of you have made out an advance directive — a living will or a health care proxy? (*It is likely that only a few people will raise their hands.*) It seems striking that, according to surveys, a great many people indicate that they approve of advance directives, but few people have actually made one out. Do you agree that advance directives are a good idea, and if so, why haven't you made one out? (*This question offers an opportunity to deal with practical issues such as to how to go about making an advance directive.*)

7. In her famous book, *On Death and Dying,* Elizabeth Kübler-Ross describes five stages in the dying or the grieving process: denial, anger, bargaining, depression, and acceptance. Can Kübler-Ross's model help us better understand the differing responses of the characters in the play? Specifically, in what stages are the Mother, the Father, and the Patient? Do any of the characters move toward "acceptance" during the play?

QUESTIONS ESPECIALLY APPROPRIATE FOR A MEDICAL AUDIENCE

1. Cases of medical futility are at present not uncommon. In your experience, what are some of the reasons behind the belief of family members that a patient will come out of such a coma?

2. Do the Patient and his parents seem realistic to you?

3. Does the Doctor respond to this situation as you would respond?

4. The play suggests some uncomfortable analogies between the Doctor and the Friend, such as the fact that both wear uniforms. Are there other similarities? In what way is a physician, like the Friend, governed by "company policy" in what he/she does or says?

5. Have you been involved in pediatric cases where the two parents disagree about the course of treatment for their child? How can we prevent parents from using their sick children as a battleground for their marital difficulties? Have you been involved in cases where adult children disagree about whether or not to remove a dying parent from life support systems? How are these cases best resolved?

6. How could communication between the parents have been facilitated? What other supports could have been brought to bear on the situation (for example, friends or religious advisors, hospital chaplains, social workers, psychologists)?

7. Most physicians have had an experience in which a "hopelessly" terminal patient recovers. This is what makes the response to the play's question, "Can you guarantee that he will never recover?" so difficult. What are some approaches to this question which you have found helpful for families grappling with this dilemma?

Appendices

A

The Values History

Patient's name: _____

This Values History serves as a set of my specific value-based directives for various medical interventions. It is to be used in health care circumstances when I may be unable to voice my preferences. These directives shall be made a part of the medical record and shall be used as supplementary to my living will and/or durable power of attorney for health care if I am terminally ill or in a persistently vegetative state.

I. *Values Section*

There are several values important in decisions about end-of-life treatment and care. This section of the Values History invites you to identify your most important values.

A. Basic Life Values

Perhaps the most basic values in this context concern length of life versus quality of life. Which of the following two statements most accurately reflects your feelings and wishes? Write your initials and the date next to the number you choose.

From David J. Doukas and L. B. McCullough, "The Values History: The Evaluation of the Patient's Values and Advance Directives," *Journal of Family Practice* 32 (1991): 143–53. Copyright © 1991 by *Journal of Family Practice,* David J. Doukas, and L. B. McCullough. Reprinted by permission of the authors, the *Journal of Family Practice* and Appleton and Lange Publishers.

_____ 1. I want to live as long as possible, regardless of the quality of life
that I experience.

_____ 2. I want to preserve a good quality of life, even if this means that I
may not live as long.

B. Quality-of-Life Values

There are many values that help us to define for ourselves the quality of life
that we want to live. The following values appear to be those most frequently used to define quality of life. Review this list and circle the values
that are most important to your definition of quality of life. Feel free to
elaborate on any of the items in the list, and to add to the list any other
values that are important to you.

1. I want to maintain my capacity to think clearly.
2. I want to feel safe and secure.
3. I want to avoid unnecessary pain and suffering.
4. I want to be treated with respect.
5. I want to be treated with dignity when I can no longer speak for
myself.
6. I do not want to be an unnecessary burden on my family.
7. I want to be able to make my own decisions.
8. I want to experience a comfortable dying process.
9. I want to be with my loved ones before I die.
10. I want to leave good memories of me for my loved ones.
11. I want to be treated in accord with my religious beliefs and
traditions.
12. I want respect shown for my body after I die.
13. I want to help others by making a contribution to medical education and research.
14. Other values or clarification of values above:

II. *Directives Section*

Some directives involve a simple yes or no decision. Others provide for the
choice of a trial of intervention. Write your initials and the date next to the
number for each directive you complete.

INITIALS / DATE

_____   1. I want to undergo cardiopulmonary resuscitation.

     _____ YES

     _____ NO

Why?

_____   2. I want to be placed on a ventilator.

     _____ YES

     _____ TRIAL for the TIME PERIOD OF _____.

     _____ TRIAL to determine effectiveness using reasonable medical judgment.

     _____ NO

Why?

_____   3. I want to have an endotracheal tube used in order to perform items 1 and 2.

     _____ YES

     _____ TRIAL for the TIME PERIOD OF _____.

     _____ TRIAL to determine effectiveness using reasonable medical judgment.

     _____ NO

Why?

_____   4. I want to have total parenteral nutrition administered for my nutrition.

     _____ YES

     _____ TRIAL for the TIME PERIOD OF _____.

     _____ TRIAL to determine effectiveness using reasonable medical judgment.

     _____ NO

Why?

_____   5. I want to have intravenous medication and hydration administered. Regardless of my decision, I understand that

intravenous hydration to alleviate discomfort or pain medication will not be withheld from me if I so request them.

_____ YES

_____ TRIAL for the TIME PERIOD OF _____.

_____ TRIAL to determine effectiveness using reasonable
medical judgment.

_____ NO

Why?

_____ 6. I want to have all medications used for the treatment of my
illness continued. Regardless of my decision, I understand
that pain medication will continue to be administered including narcotic medications.

_____ YES

_____ TRIAL for the TIME PERIOD OF _____.

_____ TRIAL to determine effectiveness using reasonable
medical judgment.

_____ NO

Why?

_____ 7. I want to have nasogastric, gastrostomy, or other enteral
feeding tubes introduced and administered for my nutrition.

_____ YES

_____ TRIAL for the TIME PERIOD OF _____.

_____ TRIAL to determine effectiveness using reasonable
medical judgment.

_____ NO

Why?

_____ 8. I want to be placed on a dialysis machine.

_____ YES

_____ TRIAL for the TIME PERIOD OF _____.

_____ TRIAL to determine effectiveness using reasonable
medical judgment.

_____ NO

Why?

_____   9. I want to have an autopsy done to determine the cause(s) of
my death.

_____ YES

_____ NO

Why?

_____   10. I want to be admitted to the Intensive Care Unit.

_____ YES

_____ NO

Why?

_____   11. *For a patient in a long-term care facility or for a patient receiving
care at home who experiences a life-threatening change in health
status:* I want 911 called in case of a medical emergency.

_____ YES

_____ NO

Why?

_____   12. Other directives:

I consent to these directives after receiving honest disclosure of their implications, risks, and benefits from my physician, being free of constraints,
and being of sound mind.

Signature: _____ Date: _____

Witness: _____

Witness: _____

13. Proxy Negation: I request that the following persons NOT be allowed
to make decisions on my behalf in the event of my disability or incapacity:

_____

_____

_____

Signature: _____ Date: _____

Witness: _____

Witness: _____

14. Organ Donation:
(Insert here your state's version of the Organ Donor Card.)

15. Durable Power of Attorney for Health Care:
(Insert here your state's version of the durable power of attorney for health care.)

B

Living Will Declaration

Declaration made this _____ day of _____, 19 ____.

A. I, _____, hereby declare and make
known to my family, physician, and others, my instructions and wishes for
my future health care. I direct that all health care decisions, including
decisions to accept or refuse any treatment, service or procedure used to
diagnose, treat or care for my physical or mental condition and decisions to
provide, withhold or withdraw life-sustaining measures, be made in accordance with my wishes as expressed in this document. This instruction
directive shall take effect in the event I become unable to make my own
health care decisions, as determined by the physician who has primary
responsibility for my care, and any necessary confirming determinations. I
direct that this document become part of my permanent medical records.

B. GENERAL INSTRUCTIONS. To inform those responsible for my
care of my specific wishes, I make the following statement of personal views
regarding my health care:

Initial ONE of the following two statements with which you agree:

1. _____ I direct that all medically appropriate measures be provided to sustain my life, regardless of my physical or mental condition.

From *A Matter of Choice: Planning Ahead for Health Care Decisions* (Washington, DC:
Health Advocacy Services of the American Association of Retired Persons, 1992), 66–68.
Copyright © 1992 by American Association of Retired Persons. Reprinted by permission.

OR

2. _____ There are circumstances in which I would not want my life to be prolonged by further medical treatment. In these circumstances, life-sustaining measures should not be initiated and if they have been, they should be discontinued. I recognize that this is likely to hasten my death. In the following, I specify the circumstances in which I would choose to forego life-sustaining measures.

If you have initialed statement 2, please intial each of the statements (a, b, c) with which you agree:

a. _____ I realize that there may come a time when I am diagnosed as having an incurable and irreversible illness, disease, or condition. If this occurs, and my attending physician and at least one additional physician who has personally examined me determine that my condition is **terminal**, I direct that life-sustaining measures which would serve only to artificially prolong my dying be withheld or discontinued. I also direct that I be given all medically appropriate care necessary to make me comfortable and to relieve pain.

b. _____ If there should come a time when I become **permanently unconscious**, and it is determined by my attending physician and at least one additional physician with appropriate expertise who has personally examined me, that I have totally and irreversibly lost consciousness and my capacity for interaction with other people and my surroundings, I direct that life-sustaining measures be withheld or discontinued. I understand that I will not experience pain or discomfort in this condition, and I direct that I be given all medically appropriate care necessary to provide for my personal hygiene and dignity.

c. _____ I realize that there may come a time when I am diagnosed as having an **incurable and irreversible** illness, disease, or condition which may not be terminal. My condition may cause me to experience severe and progressive physical or mental deterioration and/or a permanent loss of capacities and faculties I value highly. If, in the course of my medical care, the burdens of continued life with treatment become greater than the benefits I experience, I direct that life-sustaining measures be withheld or discontinued. I also direct that I be given all medically appropriate care necessary to make me comfortable and to relieve pain.

C. ADDITIONAL INSTRUCTIONS:

_____

_____

_____

_____

_____

_____

By this directive, I inform those who may become entrusted with my health care of my wishes and intend to ease the burdens of decisionmaking which this responsibility may impose. I understand the purpose and effect of this document and sign it knowingly, voluntarily and after careful deliberation.

_____
signature

_____
address

_____
city, state

WITNESSES

I declare that the person who signed this document, or asked another sign this document on his or her behalf, did so in my presence, that he or she is personally known to me, and that he or she appears to be of sound mind and free of duress or undue influence. I am at least 18 years of age and am not related to the declarant by blood or marriage, entitled to any portion of the declarant's estate under any will or by operation of law, or directly financially responsible for declarant's medical care. I am not the declarant's attending physician, an employee of the attending physician, or an employee of the health care facility in which the declarant is a patient.

1. _____
   witness

_____
address

_____
city   state

2. _____
   witness

_____
address

_____
city   state

C

Durable Power of Attorney for Health Care

1. I, _____, hereby appoint:

_____

name   home address

(_____)_____

home telephone number

(_____)_____

work telephone number

As my attorney-in-fact to make health-care decisions for me if I become unable to make my own health-care decisions. This gives my attorney-in-fact the power to grant, refuse, or withdraw consent on my behalf for any health-care service, treatment or procedure, even though my death may ensue. My attorney-in-fact has the authority to talk to health-care personnel, get information, have access to medical records, and sign forms necessary to carry out these decisions. My attorney-in-fact also has authority to authorize my admission to or discharge from any hospital, nursing home, residential care, assisted living or similar facility or service, and to contract on my behalf for any health-care related service or facility (without my attorney-in-fact incurring personal financial liability for such contracts).

2. If the person named as my attorney-in-fact is not available or is unable to act as my attorney-in-fact, I appoint the following person(s) to serve in the order listed below:

From *A Matter of Choice: Planning Ahead for Health Care Decisions* (Washington, DC: Health Advocacy Services of the American Association of Retired Persons, 1992), 66–68. Copyright © 1992 by American Association of Retired Persons. Reprinted by permission.

a. _____   _____
   name   home address

   (_____)_____
   home telephone number   _____

   (_____)_____
   work telephone number   _____

b. _____   _____
   name   home address

   (_____)_____
   home telephone number   _____

   (_____)_____
   work telephone number   _____

3.   With this document, I intend to create a durable power of attorney for health-care, which shall take effect upon and only during any period in which, in the opinion of two doctors, I am unable to make or communicate a choice regarding a particular health-care decision. My attorney-in-fact shall make health-care decisions as I direct below or as I make known to him or her in some other way. If my attorney-in-fact is unable to determine the choice I would want to make, then my attorney-in-fact shall make a choice for me based upon what my attorney-in-fact believes to be in my best interest.

a.   *STATEMENT OF DIRECTIVES CONCERNING LIFE-SUS- TAINING CARE, TREATMENT, SERVICES, AND PROCE- DURES:* (The directions herein apply to all forms of life-sustaining treatments which include but are not limited to mechanical ventilation, cardiopulmonary resuscitation, kidney dialysis, and artificial nutrition and hydration, unless otherwise limited in these directions).

_____

_____

_____

_____

_____

b. SPECIAL PROVISIONS AND LIMITATIONS: (These limitations and or provisions apply to specific types of treatment that are inconsistent with my religious beliefs or unacceptable to me for any other reason, such as blood transfusions, convulsive therapy, amputations, psychosurgery, etc., and

_____

_____

_____

_____

_____

_____

4. To the extent that I am permitted by law to do so, I herewith nominate my attorney-in-fact to serve as my guardian, conservator and/or in any similar representative capacity. If I am not permitted by law to make a nomination, then I request in the strongest possible terms that any court consider this nomination.

5. No person who relies in good faith upon representations by my attorney-in-fact or alternate attorney-in-fact shall be liable to me, my estate, my heirs or assigns for recognizing the attorney-in-fact's authority.

6. The powers delegated under this power of attorney are separable, so that the invalidity of one or more powers shall not affect any others.

BY MY SIGNATURE I INDICATE THAT I UNDERSTAND THE PURPOSE AND EFFECT OF THIS DOCUMENT.

I sign my name to this form on _____

at: _____
                    (address)

_____
         (signature)

WITNESSES

I declare that the person who signed or acknowledged this document is personally known to me, that the person signed acknowledged this durable power of attorney for health care in my presence, and that the person appears to be of sound mind and under no duress, fraud, or undue influence. I am not the person appointed as attorney-in-fact by this document, nor am I the person's health-care provider or an employee of the person's health-care provider. I am not related to the person by blood, marriage or adoption, and to the best of my knowledge, I am not a creditor of the person, nor responsible for paying the person's health-care costs, nor entitled to any part of the person's estate under a will now existing or by operation of law.

First Witness:

Signature: _____

Home Address: _____

Print Name: _____

Date: _____

Second Witness:

Signature: _____

Home Address: _____

Print Name: _____

Date: _____

NOTARIZATION

STATE OF _____) ss:

COUNTY OF _____)

    I, _____, a Notary Public in and for the
State and County aforesaid, do hereby certify that _____,
who is personally well known to me as the Principal, who executed the
foregoing Durable Power of Attorney for Health Care in said State and
County, and acknowledged that said Durable Power of Attorney for Health
Care to be the Principal's free act and voluntary deed.

    WITNESS my signature this _____ day of _____, 19_____.

_____
Notary Public

D

Resources for Consumers and Providers

Special Projects Section
American Association of Retired Persons
601 E Street NW
Washington, DC 20049 (202)434-2277

> *A Matter of Choice: Planning Ahead for Health Care Decisions* (book) — single copies at no charge
> *Tomorrow's Choices* (booklet) — single copies at no charge

American Bar Association
Commission on Legal Problems of the Elderly
1800 M Street NW, South Lobby
Washington, DC 20036 (202) 331–2297

> *Patient Self-Determination Act State Law Guide* — $5.00
> *Health Care Powers of Attorney* (booklet) — call for price

American Hospital Association
AHA Services, Inc.
P.O. Box 99376
Chicago, IL 60693 1-800-AHA-2626

> *Values in Conflict: Resolving Ethical Issues in Hospital Care* (book, #C-025002) — $20.00
> *Preparing for Advance Directives* (videotape #157301) — $500.00
> *Put It in Writing* (book, #166908) — $25.00
> *Put It in Writing* (brochure, #166909) — $12.00
> *Advance Directives: Guaranteeing Your Health Care Rights* (videotape) — $119.00

Choice in Dying (formerly Concern for Dying/Society for the Right to Die)

200 Varick Street
New York, NY 10014 (212)366-5540

> *An Act of Self-Determination* (1992; Montefiore Hospital) (videotape, 21 minutes) — $75.00
> *A Time to Choose* (1991; Albert Einstein College of Medicine) (videotape, 20 minutes) — $70.00
> *In Sickness or in Health* (1991; Montefiore Medical Center) (videotape, 33 minutes) — $75.00
> *The Right to Die: The Choice is Yours* (1987) (videotape, 14 minutes) — $38.00
> *A Good Death* (book) — $11.95
> *The Complete Guide to Living Wills* (book) — $7.95
> *Options at the End of Life* (book) — $15.00
> *Refusal-of-Treatment Legislation* (book) — $175.00
> *Case Law Fact Sheets* — $65.00
> *Maps of State Legislation* (fact sheets) — $10.00
> *Advance Directives and Community Education* (book) — $30.00

National Reference Center for Bioethics
Kennedy Institute of Ethics
Georgetown University
Washington, DC 20057 1-800-MED-ETHX

> *Living Wills and Durable Powers of Attorney: Advance Directive Legislation and Issues* (Scope Note 2) — $3.00

Center for Health Care Ethics
St. Louis University Medical Center
  Orders: Virginia Publishing
  P.O. Box 4857
  St. Louis, MO 63108 (314) 367-6612

> *Advance Directive for Future Health Care Decisions: A Christian Perspective* (booklet) — $5.00

Books on Advance Directives:

> David J. Doukas and W. Reichel, *Planning for Living Wills and Other Advance Directives for Health Care* (Baltimore: Johns Hopkins University Press, 1993).
> Norman Cantor, *Advance Directives and the Pursuit of Death with Dignity* (Bloomington: Indiana University Press, 1993).

This book has been set in Linotron Galliard. Galliard was designed for Mergenthaler in 1978 by Matthew Carter. Galliard retains many of the features of a sixteenth-century typeface cut by Robert Granjon but has some modifications that give it a more contemporary look.

Printed on acid-free paper.